100 Questions & Answers About von Willebrand Disease

Andra H. James, MD, MPH

Duke University Medical Center
Department of Hematology
Department of Obstetrics and Gynecology
Durham, North Carolina

JONES AND BARTLETT PUBLISHERS

Sudbury, Massachusetts

BOSTON   TORONTO   LONDON   SINGAPORE

World Headquarters
Jones and Bartlett Publishers
40 Tall Pine Drive
Sudbury, MA 01776
978-443-5000
info@jbpub.com
www.jbpub.com

Jones and Bartlett Publishers
Canada
6339 Ormindale Way
Mississauga, Ontario L5V 1J2
Canada

Jones and Bartlett Publishers
International
Barb House, Barb Mews
London W6 7PA
United Kingdom

Jones and Bartlett's books and products are available through most bookstores and online booksellers. To contact Jones and Bartlett Publishers directly, call 800-832-0034, fax 978-443-8000, or visit our website, www.jbpub.com.

Substantial discounts on bulk quantities of Jones and Bartlett's publications are available to corporations, professional associations, and other qualified organizations. For details and specific discount information, contact the special sales department at Jones and Bartlett via the above contact information or send an email to specialsales@jbpub.com.

The authors, editor, and publisher have made every effort to provide accurate information. However, they are not responsible for errors, omissions, or for any outcomes related to the use of the contents of this book and take no responsibility for the use of the products and procedures described. Treatments and side effects described in this book may not be applicable to all people; likewise, some people may require a dose or experience a side effect that is not described herein. Drugs and medical devices are discussed that may have limited availability controlled by the Food and Drug Administration (FDA) for use only in a research study or clinical trial. Research, clinical practice, and government regulations often change the accepted standard in this field. When consideration is being given to use of any drug in the clinical setting, the health care provider or reader is responsible for determining FDA status of the drug, reading the package insert, and reviewing prescribing information for the most up-to-date recommendations on dose, precautions, and contraindications, and determining the appropriate usage for the product. This is especially important in the case of drugs that are new or seldom used.

Production Credits
Executive Publisher: Christopher Davis
Editorial Assistant: Jessica Acox
Production Director: Amy Rose
Production Editor: Diana Coe
Associate Marketing Manager: Ilana Goddess

Manufacturing Buyer: Therese Connell
Composition: Jason Miranda/Spoke & Wheel
Cover Design: Jonathan Ayotte
Printing and Binding: Malloy, Inc.
Cover Printing: Malloy, Inc.

Cover Credits: © Dana E. Fry/ShutterStock, Inc.

Library of Congress Cataloging-in-Publication Data
James, Andra H.
  100 questions & answers about Von Willebrand disease / Andra H. James. --
1st ed.
    p. cm.
  ISBN-13: 978-0-7637-5767-0
  ISBN-10: 0-7637-5767-5
  1. Von Willebrand disease--Popular works. 2. Von Willebrand
disease--Miscellanea. I. Title. II. Title: One hundred questions & answers
about Von Willebrand disease. III. Title: 100 questions and answers about
Von Willebrand disease.
  RC647.V65J36 2009
  616.1'57--dc22
                                        2008011434
6048

Printed in the United States of America
12 11 10 09 08   10 9 8 7 6 5 4 3 2

Contents

Part 1: The Basics   *1*

Questions 1–26 cover background information, including diagnostic testing, and signs and symptoms of von Willebrand disease, with questions such as:

- How and why does blood clot?
- What is von Willebrand factor?
- What is the difference between von Willebrand disease and hemophilia?

Part 2: Treatment   *31*

Questions 27–54 explore a number of options to treat VWD and to help control bleeding, including:

- How is von Willebrand factor replaced?
- What are topical agents and how can they help?
- What if I have to have an operation or other procedure? How is bleeding prevented?

Part 3: Women's Issues   *55*

Questions 55–76 address concerns specifically targeted to women with VWD, such as:

- How is menorrhagia or heavy menstrual bleeding managed?
- What are hemorrhagic cysts?
- Is treatment of VWD safe for an unborn baby?
- What is a normal amount of bleeding after childbirth?

Part 4: Managing Other Bleeding Symptoms   *77*

Questions 77–84 discuss a variety of other bleeding symptoms that may occur, including:

- What if there is blood in my urine?
- What if I get a nosebleed?
- Can von Willebrand disease cause joint bleeds?

Part 5: Living with VWD 89

Questions 85–100 provide practical advice regarding lifestyle choices and how they will affect your VWD, such as:

- Are there medications that I should avoid?
- Does eating foods high in vitamin K prevent bleeding?
- Is a medical identification bracelet necessary?

Foreword

In von Willebrand disease (VWD), low or absent levels of the blood protein, von Willebrand factor, affect the blood's ability to clot. Von Willebrand factor carries with it clotting factor VIII, another important protein that helps blood clot. Von Willebrand disease is typically milder, but more common than another clotting disorder, hemophilia. For some people with VWD, however, the condition can pose serious health risks, especially during surgery, following an injury, or during childbirth. Von Willebrand disease affects 1 out of every 100 to 10,000 people—both males and females—whereas hemophilia affects mainly males. There is no one test for the disease, and it is difficult to diagnose.

Both individuals with the condition and their physicians often fail to recognize that a bleeding disorder is present. Consequently, when individuals who are unaware of their condition face bleeding challenges, they are at risk of having a hemorrhage.

Ideally, individuals recognize their bleeding symptoms and report them to their physicians. Physicians should take a complete medical history, perform a physical examination, and order a sequence of blood tests to evaluate persons whose symptoms suggest VWD or any bleeding disorder. The symptoms of VWD include frequent large bruises from minor bumps or injuries, frequent or hard-to-stop nosebleeds, extended bleeding from the gums after dental procedures, heavy bleeding after a cut or after surgery, and heavy menstrual bleeding in women. People with type 1 or type 2 VWD may not have major bleeding problems and, as a result, may not be diagnosed until they have heavy bleeding after surgery or some other bleeding challenge. In contrast, type 3 VWD can cause major bleeding problems during infancy and childhood. As a result, children with type 3 VWD are usually diagnosed during their first year of life. Although VWD cannot be cured, it can be treated. Proper diagnosis is important, and with the right treatment plan, even people with type 3 VWD, the most serious form, can live long, healthy, active lives.

Treatment for VWD depends on its type and severity, and this is why it is important to know the type of VWD a person has. Most cases of VWD are mild and may require treatment only for surgery, tooth extraction, or injury. Medicines may be prescribed to replace von Willebrand factor or increase the release of it into the bloodstream (desmopressin or DDAVP), to prevent the breakdown of clots (anti-fibrinolytics), or to control heavy menstrual bleeding in women (the hormones estrogen and progestin).

It is important for people with VWD to avoid over-the-counter medicines that can affect blood clotting, including aspirin, ibuprofen, and other nonsteroidal anti-inflammatory drugs (NSAIDs). Those with VWD should talk to their dentist to determine if medicine is needed before dental work to reduce bleeding, and anyone over two years of age with VWD should be immunized against hepatitis A and B to minimize the potential for contracting a virus with transfusions. It is important for individuals with VWD to exercise regularly and maintain a healthy weight. Safe exercises include swimming, biking, and walking. Sports that carry a higher likelihood of injury, such as football, hockey, wrestling, and lifting heavy weights, are not recommended for people with VWD.

This book covers many of these important issues in detail. One hundred different questions are answered that cover basic information, treatment, women's issues, and management of bleeding symptoms. The book does a nice job of incorporating individuals' stories in a way that highlights and personalizes the answers to the questions. It is an excellent resource not only for individuals with VWD but for others who would like to learn more about the condition.

Thomas L. Ortel, MD, PhD
Director, Duke Comprehensive Hemostasis and Thrombosis Center
Professor of Medicine, Duke University

Introduction

I was compelled to write this book, *100 Questions & Answers About von Willebrand Disease*, because I wanted a resource to share with my patients and their families. None of the information in this book is new or original, and all of it is available in other books, articles, and Web sites, but I wanted the information assembled in one place so I could hand it to my patients and their families. When I mentioned the possibility of creating such a book to my contacts within the bleeding disorders community, I was met with enthusiasm. I approached Chris Davis, executive publisher at Jones and Bartlett. He endorsed the concept and agreed to publish the book.

The book has answers to 100 questions concerning basic information, treatment, women's issues, and management of bleeding symptoms for individuals with von Willebrand disease. I have answered the questions using conversational English as opposed to medical terms, and where I have used medical terms, I have defined and explained them. Each question and answer can be read individually, so that the book can be used as a reference and also read in its entirety, if desired.

The questions in the book have been culled not only from encounters with patients and their families but from consumers at "Ask the Expert" sessions and "Rap Sessions" held at the National Hemophilia Foundation (NHF) annual meeting and at "NHF On the Road" outreach programs. The answers have come from my experience, my work in the field, my colleagues in the United States and abroad, and from my fellow panel members on the National Heart, Lung, and Blood Institute's von Willebrand Disease Expert Panel. The National Heart, Lung, and Blood Institute and the panel produced the United States' first national guidelines on von Willebrand disease. The final document, *The Diagnosis, Evaluation, and Management of von Willebrand Disease*, was released on February 29, 2008. I am indebted to my fellow panel members—William L. Nichols, Jr, MD, Chair; Mae B. Hultin, MD; Marilyn J. Manco-Johnson, MD; Robert R. Montgomery, MD; Thomas L. Ortel, MD, PhD; Margaret E. Rick, MD; J. Evan Sadler, MD, PhD; Mark Weinstein, PhD; and Barbara P. Yawn, MD, MSc; as well as the National Heart, Lung, and Blood Institute staff members—Barbara Link, PhD, and Sue Rogus, RN, MS, for the opportunity to serve with them and learn from them.

My path to becoming an advocate for women with bleeding disorders began with the delivery of a woman with factor II, VII, IX, and X deficiency, otherwise known as Borgschulte–Grigsbee deficiency. She was the first person to be described with this condition. Her maiden name happened to be Borgschulte. I was profoundly moved by the bleeding she experienced. Since then, I have sought to learn as much as possible about caring for individuals with bleeding disorders.

During my fellowship in maternal-fetal medicine, I spent two years in the laboratory of Russell Ware, MD, PhD, who invited me to join him and the rest of the laboratory staff in attending the American Society of Hematology meeting in Miami in December 1998. It was there that I attended a seminar sponsored by Centeon, one of the forerunners of CSL Behring. I heard giants in the field of women's bleeding disorders—Jean Lusher, MD, Stephanie Seremetis, MD, Christine Lee, MD, and Rezan Kadir, MD—expound on the subject. I would like to think that after that seminar, I began to follow in their footsteps. An interesting twist occurred—after returning from the meeting, I began testing women with menorrhagia for von Willebrand disease and learned that I had a mild form of the disease myself.

In 2000, with the blessing of my division director, R. Phillip Heine, MD, I formalized a clinic for women with bleeding and clotting disorders, which became a part of a larger Comprehensive Hemostasis and Thrombosis Center at Duke. In 2001, we received funding from the Centers for Disease Control and Prevention's Division of Blood

Disorders for our center. During a site visit by their staff, I met Sally Owens, RN She introduced me to the wonderful and dedicated staff at the NHF. As a member of the Women's Task Force, I continue to work closely with Ann Marie Nazzaro, Vice President for Education, and Anna DeSimone, Director of Education, and am inspired by their indefatigable efforts on behalf of individuals with bleeding disorders.

I must also thank the Centers for Disease Control and Prevention's Blood Disorders Division for continuing to fund research in women's bleeding disorders and for introducing me to two of my current research collaborators—Claire Philipp, MD, and Peter Kouides, MD My other research collaborator in women's bleeding disorders is Barbara Konkle, MD, who now chairs the NHF's Women's Task Force.

I am always supported in my work with women and bleeding disorders by our staff in the Women's Hemostasis and Thrombosis Clinic—our nurses, Kim Adcock, Geri Wahlay, Melissa Britt, and Lynn Britt; our genetic counselor, Kristin Nuñez; my partner, Leo R. Brancazio, MD; our maternal-fetal medicine fellows; and our selfless and dedicated project coordinator, Betty Thames.

In preparing the book, I have been inspired by my patients, their family members, and others whom I have met in the bleeding disorders community. Some have graciously shared their stories in this book. They are:
- Judi Miller, Vice President of Medical Affairs at Octapharma, USA, Inc.
- Jessica Acox, Editorial Assistant, Jones and Bartlett Publishers
- Jeanette, CPA and Business Management Consultant
- Vicki Pratt-Jacobs, Maine Program and Red Flag of New England Coordinator
- Nikki Rickard, mother and grandmother
- Gary McKissick, mechanic
- Ray Pierce, student at the Catholic University of America
- Karen Anderson, writer and mother

In preparing this book, I was encouraged by my mentor and colleague, Dr. Thomas L. Ortel, hematologist and Director of our Duke Comprehensive Hemostasis and Thrombosis Center, who answers my patient-related questions no matter what time of day or night it is. He is a superb doctor and patient human being. He also graciously agreed to write the foreword.

I would like to dedicate this book to all of my patients, coworkers, colleagues, collaborators, and friends in the bleeding disorders community. They have all made it possible.

Andra H. James, MD, MPH

PART ONE

The Basics

How and why does blood clot?

What is von Willebrand factor?

What is the difference between
von Willebrand disease and hemophilia?

More . . .

1. What is blood?

Blood, a fluid that transports essential substances around the body, is composed of water, proteins, other molecules, and cells. The main type of cell in the blood is the red blood cell. Red blood cells contain **hemoglobin**, a molecule that has the unique ability to pick up oxygen in areas of the body where the concentration of oxygen is high (the lungs), carry it to other parts of the body, and release it where the concentration of oxygen is low (arms, legs, and organs other than the lungs). Oxygen combines with energy sources derived from food to provide "fuel" to individual cells within the tissue of organs and extremities so that the cells can survive and function. In the process, carbon dioxide is produced and must be carried away. Hemoglobin also has the ability to pick up carbon dioxide where the concentration of carbon dioxide is high (arms, legs, and organs other than the lungs) and release it where the concentration is low (the lungs). Therefore, the purpose of red blood cells is to carry oxygen to the cells within the tissue of organs and extremities (arms and legs) and carry carbon dioxide away. The other types of cells in blood are white blood cells and **platelets**. White blood cells fight infections. Platelets help prevent blood from leaking out of injured **blood vessels**.

The liquid portion of blood that contains proteins and other molecules, but does not include cells, is called **plasma**. Plasma, which is 90% water, constitutes 55% of blood volume. Plasma contains albumin (the chief protein constituent), fibrinogen (a specialized protein or **clotting factor**), and globulins (including antibodies). Plasma serves as the medium of exchange for essential minerals such as sodium and potassium, helping maintain a proper balance in the body, which is critical to cell

Blood

A fluid that transports essential substances around the body and is composed of water, proteins, other molecules, and cells.

Hemoglobin

The molecule in the red blood cells that carries oxygen in the blood and gives blood its red color.

Platelets

The cells that prevent blood from leaking out of injured blood vessels.

Blood vessels

Tubes that carry blood to organs and extremities.

Plasma

The liquid portion of blood that contains proteins and other molecules, but does not include cells.

Clotting factor

A specialized protein that is essential to prevent bleeding.

function. It also serves a variety of other functions, from maintaining a satisfactory blood pressure and volume to supplying critical proteins for immunity (antibodies) and blood coagulation (clotting factors).

2. What are blood vessels?

Blood vessels are the tubes that carry blood to organs and extremities. There are two major types of blood vessels—arteries and veins. Arteries are thick, muscular vessels that carry blood away from the heart. Within organs and extremities, arteries branch into smaller vessels called arterioles, and arterioles branch into capillaries. Capillaries are thin, tiny vessels that allow molecules, fluids, and even some cells to travel in and out of them. The capillaries branch into larger blood vessels called venules, and venules branch into veins. Veins carry blood back to the heart from organs and extremities.

There are two major types of blood vessels—arteries and veins.

Blood returns from organs and extremities to the right side of the heart through a very large vein called the vena cava. The right side of the heart, particularly the right ventricle, pumps blood through a very large artery, the pulmonary artery, to the lungs. Inside the lungs, the pulmonary artery branches into smaller arterioles and the even smaller capillaries. Carbon dioxide passes out of the capillaries into the air sacs (alveoli) of the lungs, and simultaneously oxygen passes out of the alveoli into the capillaries. The newly oxygenated blood travels from the capillaries through the venules and pulmonary veins into the left side of the heart, where it is pumped by the left ventricle through a very large artery, the aorta, to the rest of the body.

3. How and why does blood clot?

Since normal blood flow is necessary to supply oxygen to organs and extremities and to carry carbon dioxide away, damage to a blood vessel or blood vessels could jeopardize life-sustaining functions by allowing blood to leak out. Therefore, all animals, including humans, have an inborn mechanism to plug a possible leak at the site of blood vessel injury. This mechanism is called blood clotting or coagulation.

Blood vessels can be injured in many ways including minor trauma, serious injuries, surgery, or disease. Ordinarily, blood vessels are lined by a smooth, slippery surface called the **endothelium**. When blood vessels are injured, the endothelium is damaged and the tissue underneath the endothelium, the **subendothelium**, is exposed. The subendothelium, composed of the protein collagen, is rough and sticky. Platelets, the cells that prevent blood from leaking out of an injured blood vessel, stick or adhere to the subendothelium where it is exposed. In the process, the platelets change shape from a disk shape to a globular shape like an ameba. While the platelets are changing shape, certain internal structures or granules are disrupted and release substances that activate the platelets. Activated platelets have receptors on their surfaces that allow them to stick to one another or aggregate. Aggregated platelets form a plug at the site of a possible leak.

The plug is just a clump of platelets it is held in place by a mesh or net made of a substance called **fibrin**. Fibrin is solid and is formed from fibrinogen, a specialized protein or clotting factor that is found in blood. When a blood vessel is injured, the exposed subendothelium allows a protein known as tissue factor to be exposed to

Endothelium

The lining of blood vessels.

Subendothelium

The tissue under the endothelium, which is the lining of the blood vessels. Platelets, the cells that prevent blood from leaking out of an injured blood vessel, stick or adhere to the subendothelium.

Fibrin

A solid mesh or net formed from fibrinogen, a specialized protein or clotting factor. Fibrin holds platelets and other cells in place and prevents blood from leaking out of an injured blood vessel.

the blood. Tissue factor sets off a chain reaction, called the coagulation cascade, that activates a whole series of clotting factors. The last step of this chain reaction is the conversion of fibrinogen into fibrin, which forms the mesh or net that holds the platelets firmly in place, forming a clot. The clot, therefore, is made up of fibrin, platelets, and other cells, particularly red blood cells that are trapped in the process.

4. What is von Willebrand factor?

Von Willebrand factor (VWF) is a protein that is essential for normal blood clotting. It acts like a glue to stick or adhere platelets to the subendothelium at the site of blood vessel injury. Not only does VWF adhere platelets to subendothelium, but it helps platelets attach to one another, or aggregate, and protects one of the clotting factors, **factor VIII**, from being destroyed in the circulation. Von Willebrand factor is formed from identical subunits that are produced inside of endothelial cells and assembled into strings of varying size called **von Willebrand factor multimers**. Once assembled, VWF multimers are stored within packets or granules called Weibel-Palade bodies. Von Willebrand factor is also present in platelets.

5. What is von Willebrand disease?

Von Willebrand disease (VWD) is a bleeding tendency resulting from insufficient or low levels of VWF, abnormal VWF, or absent VWF. Although VWD cannot be cured, the risk of bleeding can be reduced and the condition can be treated. For most people with VWD, the condition is mild and manageable.

von Willebrand factor (VWF)

A protein that is essential for normal blood clotting. It acts like a glue to stick or adhere platelets to the subendothelium at the site of blood vessel injury.

Factor VIII

One of the clotting factors that is essential to prevent bleeding.

von Willebrand factor multimers

Strings of von Willebrand subunits that form the active forms of von Willebrand factor.

von Willebrand disease (VWD)

A bleeding tendency resulting from insufficient or low levels of von Willebrand, abnormal von Willebrand factor, or absent von Willebrand factor.

While VWD cannot be cured, the risk of bleeding can be reduced and the condition can be treated.

Andra's story (low VWF or mild type 1 VWD):

I trained as an obstetrician gynecologist at the University of North Carolina in Chapel Hill, which is renowned for research on the treatment of hemophilia. While I was there, I developed an interest in the care of women with bleeding and clotting disorders. Actually, my interest was sparked by one particular woman, a woman with deficiencies of blood clotting factors II, VII, IX, and X. Before I trained as an obstetrician gynecologist, I worked as a nurse-midwife and had delivered approximately 1,000 babies before I ever went to medical school. I had come to rely on normal blood clotting at the time of delivery. When I delivered the woman with factor II, VII, IX, and X deficiency, I got a surprise. While her uterus contracted, and she had no more than the usual amount of bleeding from it, she began to hemorrhage from the simple episiotomy (incision to enlarge the vaginal opening) I had made to allow the delivery of her 9 pound, 12 ounce baby. No amount of pressure would stop the bleeding, and it was not until she had received three units of fresh frozen plasma that the bleeding subsided. I was profoundly moved by what I had observed and was compelled to learn as much as I could about the role of blood clotting factors in women's health.

After my training, I went to Duke University to do a fellowship in maternal-fetal medicine (high-risk obstetrics). All of the maternal-fetal medicine faculty and senior fellows knew more about just about everything in high-risk obstetrics than I did, except bleeding and clotting. My reading and my training at Chapel Hill had provided me with an advantage in caring for women with bleeding and clotting disorders and I began to see women with these problems in my clinic. Halfway through my first year of fellowship, I decided that I would spend my mandatory research time on a project related to blood clotting. I approached Dr. Russell Ware, a pediatric hematologist, and he welcomed me into his lab. The following year, he invited me to accompany him and the rest of the lab staff to a meeting of the American Society of Hematology. While I was there, I attended a seminar about bleeding disorders in women. One of the presenters said that every woman with heavy menstrual bleeding should be tested for a bleeding disorder. I was shocked! Throughout my training, all the women I met with bleeding disorders had already been diagnosed. I had never encountered a woman with heavy menstrual bleeding who was later found to have a bleeding disorder. Or had I and I didn't know it?

Coincidentally, just a few weeks after I returned from the meeting, I was approached by a company that makes a platelet function analyzer. The platelet function analyzer, the PFA-100®, has been found to detect a high percentage of cases of von Willebrand disease. The company asked me if I knew how their instrument might be useful in women's health. I remembered what the presenter at the American Society of Hematology meeting had said, that every woman with heavy menstrual bleeding should be tested for a bleeding disorder, and proposed to the company that we use the platelet function analyzer to test women with heavy menstrual bleeding and look for von Willebrand disease. The company accepted the proposal and we began the study at our institution. We were surprised to learn that even among women who had no confirmation other than a physician diagnosis of menorrhagia (heavy menstrual bleeding), 6 percent were ultimately found to have von Willebrand disease, and among white women, the rate was even higher: 10 percent.

One of the women who enrolled in the study had seen her physician two years earlier and told her physician that she had "heavy periods, just like [her] mother." That should have raised a red flag, but apparently it didn't. While she was awaiting a hysterectomy to treat her heavy, painful periods, her husband learned about our study. He told her he thought she had von Willebrand disease and should enroll in our study, so she did. As it turned out, she had a von Willebrand factor level of less than 50 percent of normal and was diagnosed with mild type 1 von Willebrand disease, or what, alternately, we would now call low von Willebrand factor. One of the ironies of this story is that her physician was my co-investigator on the study, but the bigger irony is that I was the patient. It took my husband, who is an engineer and not a doctor, to recognize my tendency to bleed.

Since then, I have reflected on my condition. I honestly used to believe that my tendency to bleed was normal and judged my patients accordingly. When I was in training, if a woman came to me with heavy menstrual bleeding but described bleeding similar to my own, I reassured her that that was normal. If someone complained about easy bruising, I was unimpressed. If someone oozed from her surgical wounds, I found that within the range of normal. I now recognize that I do tend to bleed more than the average person. In fact, my husband, who takes the blood thinner Coumadin® because of his history of abnormal blood clots, does not bleed as easily as I do. On the other hand, I am only mildly affected; I do not experience spontaneous bleeding and do not have to be concerned about my condition except when I am getting ready to have surgery. This is not true for individuals who are moderately or severely affected and are much more likely to bleed than I am. I have learned from them, as well as myself, that there is a wide range of bleeding tendencies with von Willebrand disease, that von Willebrand factor levels do not always predict bleeding tendencies, that each individual is different and that even in the same individual, different situations may provoke a different amount of bleeding.

6. Who discovered VWD?

Von Willebrand disease was first described in 1926 by Erik von Willebrand, a Finnish physician and professor of medicine at the University of Helsinki. Although he wrote articles about a number of medical subjects, he is most famous for his description of the disease that bears his name. In his original paper on VWD, he noted that bleeding manifestations were more likely to involve mucosal surfaces as opposed to joints, which is the case with **hemophilia**. The first patient in his report was a 5-year-old girl from the Åland islands who had already lost three siblings to the disease. Her mother's maternal grandmother had bled to death in childbirth, and the patient herself ultimately bled to death during her fourth menstrual period. Dr. von Willebrand examined 66 members of the patient's family and found that 23 had a bleeding disorder—16 females and 7 males. Previously, hereditary hemorrhagic disease had been regarded as synonymous with hemophilia, a disease primarily of males, but in his series of cases, women appeared to be twice as likely to be affected as men.

Hemophilia

A severe bleeding disorder that results from a deficiency of clotting factor VIII (hemophilia A) or clotting factor IX (hemophilia B).

7. What are the signs and symptoms of VWD?

The signs and symptoms of VWD depend on the type and severity of the disease. Many people have such mild symptoms that they do not know they have the disease. Signs and symptoms of VWD usually involve abnormal bleeding from the skin and mucous membranes (the lining of the nose, mouth, intestines, uterus, and vagina). Most people with VWD have type 1 disease. They have bleeding that is mild to moderate in severity, does not require routine transfusions or other treatments, and is not life threatening. Life-threatening

Many people have such mild symptoms that they do not know they have the disease.

bleeding involving the brain or intestines can occur in individuals with type 3 disease, in some individuals with type 2 disease, and rarely in individuals with type 1 disease. Bleeding within deep tissues, such as muscles and joints, may occur in individuals with type 3 disease. Other medical conditions such as liver or kidney disease and medications including aspirin, nonsteroidal anti-inflammatory drugs, and anticoagulants can make the bleeding tendency worse. The following are specific signs and symptoms of VWD:

- Prolonged bleeding from trivial wounds, lasting more than 15 minutes or recurring spontaneously during the 7 days after the wound

- Heavy, prolonged, or recurrent bleeding after surgery such as a tonsillectomy

- Bruising with minimal or no trauma, especially bruising resulting in a lump

- Nosebleeds that last more than 10 minutes or require medical attention to stop

- Heavy, prolonged, or recurrent bleeding after dental procedures or tooth extraction

- Unexplained bleeding from the stomach or intestines

- Anemia requiring iron therapy or transfusion

- Heavy menstrual bleeding requiring more than one pad or tampon in an hour's period of time or resulting in clots an inch in diameter or more in size

Judi's story (moderate type 1 VWD):

As a young girl growing up it was always my job to clean the bathroom. "Why me?" I would ask.

"Because you mess it up . . . there's always blood in the sink after you've been in there," the family would respond.

Fast forward a few years to the start of menstruation . . . or, as it was better known in my house, "the curse." My mom, thoroughly modern, had warned me what to expect . . . though she never referred to it as bleeding, always as flooding. And she was right. From the first period I was using tampons and pads together . . . lots of them, just as she had always done.

Around the same time, I remember reading in a magazine that women lost an average of three teaspoons of blood per period. I just dismissed this, thinking it must be a typo or gross underexaggeration so as not to frighten young girls.

Not knowing any better, I wasn't concerned other than that the bleeding interfered with my sport, in particular gymnastics and badminton. Keeping regulation "whites" white was somewhat of a challenge. I guess it was this that made me discuss the bleeding with my family doctor. He agreed the bleeding was excessive and prescribed "the pill," but told me that as I was only 13, I should never tell anyone about this!

With my periods more or less under control, my next challenge was nosebleeds. I'd always had them, but they became more frequent—two to three per day, usually profuse enough for the teachers to throw me out of class before fellow students fainted.

Although this was a great excuse for avoiding everyday math and German lessons, with major exams looming, it was off to the doctor again.

A botched bilateral cauterization procedure left me with embarrassing black burns under my nostrils, but helped with the nosebleeds.

A tonsillectomy at 18 was complicated by severe post-op bleeding as was a routine D & C procedure a few years later. Being rushed back in over a weekend and ending up in my own hospital for emergency packing and transfusion was somewhat humiliating and inconvenient, but nothing more than "one of those things."

Despite these minor setbacks, my career took off successfully and I frequently found myself lecturing at medical conferences around the world.

I was honored to be an invited speaker at the first ever Congress on Bleeding Disorders and Transfusion Medicine in South America. Relaxing around the pool, in Punta del Este, Uruguay, ahead of my lecture on VWD, I found myself next to some former associates from London. After exchanging the usual pleasantries and catching up on gossip, one of them, an eminent hemophilia specialist, asked me how the other guy was doing. Somewhat confused, I asked him what he meant.

"Your legs," he explained, "they're covered in bruises."

"Oh, it's nothing, they're always like that," I replied.

A few probing questions and several blood tests later, I was diagnosed with moderate type 1 VWD.

With the benefit of hindsight this should of course have been picked up earlier . . . if not by one of the many doctors that I saw, then by self-diagnosis.

How many times had I lectured on women's bleeding disorders over the years? How many times had I spoken the words that VWD is the most underdiagnosed bleeding disorder? How stupid did I feel?

What I now realize is that my mother also has VWD. She saw nothing unusual in my heavy periods, having always suffered from them herself. Bruising and gum bleeds were part of her life too. My grandmother was almost certainly affected. One of my earliest memories is of her almost hemorrhaging to death when her femoral artery spontaneously ruptured.

I still bleed, I still have bruises, but I consider myself one of the lucky ones. Knowing that I have a bleeding disorder allows me to make smarter choices and may even save my life one day. I now share my story in lectures in the hope that others will be diagnosed earlier.

Jessica's story (type 1 VWD):

I wasn't diagnosed with VWD until my freshman year of high school. I had always had bloody noses when I was grow-ing up, but nothing that my family thought was unusual. My mom even later admitted that she had assumed that I was a kid who aggressively picked her nose (thanks Mom!). Preceding my diagnosis, I had had four bloody noses within a week's time, and all had a heavy flow for over 45 minutes. I believe the longest was pushing an hour and 15 minutes. We finally went to the emergency room, where they took blood and performed a barrage of tests. At the time, the diagnosis was surprising—most likely because we had never heard of VWD before, nor were we expecting any news like that— although looking back on it, it makes a lot of sense. I bruised easily, had an abnormal period, and was anemic.

Jeanette's story (type 1 VWD with a platelet defect):

I always knew we were free bleeders; that was just the way it was; but I wasn't diagnosed until I was 20 or 25 years old, and even then, it was because I was a ward secretary at the Jamaica Plain Veterans Hospital and was able to participate in a study while still getting paid for the time I was away from my desk. A doctor there was doing research, and he found out that my blood was different! He told me I had VWD. He studied me for six months. I still have scars up and down my arms from all the bleeding times that were done. He had my parents come in. My mother had VWD, too. My father, as it turned out, had some kind of platelet defect. Even now, my diagnosis is still uncertain. My children and I have had some strange test results and are undergoing additional tests. As it turns out, we may have some type of type 2 VWD along with platelet dysfunction.

My first bleed was when I had my tonsils out at age 6. Although some might not agree, two days later was the best day of my life. I got a lot of attention. It was a Sunday and all of my Irish Catholic family was having dinner at our house in our small town on the South Shore of Boston. I was forced to sit at the table with the family, but I felt sick. Eventually, I felt so bad that I had to go upstairs and throw up. When I threw up, blood began pouring out of my mouth. My parents called the ambulance. A police car arrived before the ambulance did. A police officer, whom I recognized (like I said, it was a small town and we knew everyone), carried me out to his car. I felt no pain, maybe because I was ready to faint. I remember floating up and watching the police car speeding through the streets. When we got to the hospital, I remember the nurse putting needles in, but I still felt no pain. The first time I realized that something was wrong was when my father collapsed and started crying. I was transfused a lot of blood.

I feel bad now, because the surgeon was blamed. We must have received some sort of compensation, because I remember that we got a new TV. We didn't realize that there was a bleeding problem in the family.

Different types of VWD require different treatment, so knowing the type of VWD is important.

---

8. What are the differences between types 1, 2, and 3 VWD?

Different types of VWD require different treatment, so knowing the type of VWD is important. Type 1, the most common type of VWD, is characterized by low levels of

VWF and is usually mild. Type 2 VWD is characterized by abnormal VWF. There are four subtypes:

- Type 2A is characterized by a deficiency of normal multimers of VWF.

- Type 2B is characterized by VWF that binds too tightly to platelets and can result in a low number of platelets or thrombocytopenia.

- Type 2M is characterized by VWF that does not bind tightly enough to platelets.

- Type 2N is characterized by VWF that does not bind well to factor VIII and therefore does not protect factor VIII from being destroyed in the circulation. Because factor VIII levels are low, individuals with type 2N VWD resemble individuals with factor VIII deficiency or hemophilia A.

Type 3 VWD is characterized by the virtual absence of von Willebrand factor and is usually severe.

Vicki's story (type 3 VWD):

I started showing symptoms of a bleeding disorder in 1958 at six weeks old with bruises on my chest and the back of my head. I was put through the whole gamut of testing that Maine could offer at the time, including a lumbar puncture (to test for leukemia), which I nearly died from. The pediatrician told my mom that he would know exactly what I had, had I been a boy—hemophilia!! They knew of a well-known hematologist in Boston that ran a specialty clinic for bleeding disorders and referred me down to that clinic. I was diagnosed with von Willebrand disease in 1960, at the age of 18 months, by Dr. Diamond at Boston Children's Hospital. At that time, only a handful of people had been diagnosed, and family studies were done to track heredity patterns.

In 1992, I got sick again with the lightheadedness that by this time I knew to be anemia. I let it go for several days and then could not ignore it any longer. Off to the doctor I went. . . . The doctor determined that I was having some bleeding in my gastrointestinal tract and I had lost a lot of blood. I was admitted to the military hospital where my husband was stationed. At the hospital, they gave me a transfusion of two units of whole blood and discussed my situation with a hematologist outside the military hospital. Soon I was moved from the military hospital to a hospital downtown. The hematologist took the customary eight vials of blood, which he in turn sent to the Mayo Clinic in Minnesota for evaluation. The results returned a verdict of type 3 VWD with levels less than 12% of normal. I did not even know that VWD had types. The doctor told me that there was a treatment [with a VWF/FVIII concentrate] to be used in a life-or-death situation and, with respect to treatment, that I should carry on doing what I had been doing in the past, which, until that time, was nothing.

Nikki's story (type 2B VWD):

I was diagnosed with type 2B VWD after I fell and broke my leg. I had an epidural anesthetic for the repair and developed an epidural hematoma. My platelets were low, but not low enough, in the opinion of my orthopedic surgeon, to explain an epidural hematoma (a very rare complication of an epidural anesthetic, but one that can cause temporary or even permanent paralysis). I was very fortunate that in my case the paralysis was temporary. My orthopedic surgeon sent me to a hematologist who thought my low platelets were no big deal. My orthopedic surgeon was not satisfied with that explanation and sent me to a specialist in bleeding disorders at Stanford University. The specialist took one look at my blood under the microscope and recognized a problem instantly, but had me come back three times for additional tests before he was able to make the diagnosis of type 2B VWD.

When my youngest daughter was 16 years old, she played soccer. Even though this is a contact sport, she was flexible and coordinated, so I was surprised by the large bruises she would get. One day her coach called me because she thought my daughter was sick and might have mono. I took her to the doctor, who found out that my daughter did not have mono, but her platelet count was very low (40,000). The doctor told me that my daughter did not have VWD.

After my daughter went away to college in Boston at age 17, my hematologist strongly recommended that she be tested. My daughter was seen at the Dana-Farber Cancer Institute, but they did not diagnose her with VWD. When she came home for the summer, I was still concerned that she had VWD and took her to Stanford, where she was finally diagnosed with type 2B VWD. While she was there, she was also found to be severely anemic. She had started having her periods just a year earlier and was hemorrhaging with every one. She responded well to hormones and has not required any VWF concentrates. In retrospect, she had a gastric bleed as a baby, which should have raised our suspicions that she had a bleeding disorder.

Since then, two of my other daughters and two of my grandchildren have been diagnosed with type 2B VWD. When one of these daughters was diagnosed at Stanford, a fellow in hematology was visiting from Montreal who knew of an extended family, descended from Norman French and living in Quebec, who had type 2B VWD. Their name was Paquet. We were amazed. My maiden name was Paquet.

9. What is acquired VWD or acquired von Willebrand syndrome (AVWS)?

Von Willebrand disease is usually inherited, but in rare cases, it can be acquired over the course of an individual's lifetime

Von Willebrand disease is usually inherited, but in rare cases, it can be acquired over the course of an individual's lifetime as a result of another medical condition.

as a result of another medical condition. This is called acquired von Willebrand syndrome (AVWS). Sometimes AVWS can result from specific immune proteins or antibodies that attack von Willebrand factor. These antibodies may be present in an autoimmune disorder, such as lupus, in which antibodies are made against an individual's own tissues; disorders of blood production (myeloproliferative disorders); and certain cancers. Sometimes AVWS can result from damage to von Willebrand factor multimers from abnormal heart valves or other heart defects. Sometimes AVWS can result from thyroid disease, specifically hypothyroidism, which is characterized by low levels of thyroid hormone. Correction of low thyroid levels with thyroid medication restores normal production of VWF and eliminates the AVWS.

10. How is VWD inherited?

Autosomal dominant transmission

The mode of inheritance when there is an abnormal gene on one of the chromosomes among the 22 pairs of autosomes, or non—sex (X or Y) chromosomes. Only one of the parents will have the condition caused by the abnormal gene. Only one parent needs to have the abnormal gene for the condition to be transmitted.

With the exception of type 3 VWD, which is rare and severe, and cases of type 2N VWD, VWD is generally inherited by **autosomal dominant transmission**. Autosomal dominant transmission occurs when there is an abnormal gene on one of the chromosomes among the 22 pairs of autosomes, or non—sex (X or Y) chromosomes. Since the condition is dominant, as opposed to recessive, only one of the parents will have the condition caused by the abnormal gene. Only one parent needs to have the abnormal gene for the condition to be transmitted. Therefore, conditions with autosomal dominant transmission are present in every generation. Because the abnormal gene is on an autosome, as opposed to one of the sex chromosomes, males and females are equally likely to have the condition. Each affected individual has an affected parent, and each affected individual has a 50% chance of transmitting the condition to his or her child. Individuals without the condition do not transmit the condition. Exceptions to this pattern of inheritance can occur when a new mutation or abnormality in a gene occurs, when mild forms of the condition are overlooked, or when other factors determine whether symptoms are present. In theory, women and girls are no more likely to inherit VWD than men and boys, but Erik von Willebrand found that females were twice as likely to be affected as males. This is likely a reflection of the fact that the condition may be overlooked in men and boys, while women and girls experience bleeding with menstruation and childbirth.

Type 3 VWD and cases of type 2N VWD are inherited by **autosomal recessive transmission**. Autosomal recessive transmission occurs when there is an abnormal gene on both chromosomes in a pair of the 22 pairs of autosomes, or non–sex (X or Y) chromosomes. Autosomal recessive diseases, like type 3 VWD and some cases of type 2 VWD, are rare. For an individual to be affected, he or she has to inherit the abnormal gene from both parents. The affected individual has no normal gene and consequently has a much more severe form of a disease than someone with only one abnormal gene.

Autosomal recessive transmission

The mode of inheritance when there is an abnormal gene on both chromosomes in a pair of the 22 pairs of autosomes, or non–sex (X or Y) chromosomes.

Because VWD is inherited and can be transmitted, individuals with VWD and their family members should have the opportunity to meet with a knowledgeable genetic counselor.

Garry's story (type 2A VWD):
My daughter inherited von Willebrand disease from me. My two sisters and I inherited it from my father. My father inherited it from his father. When I was growing up, I knew we were free bleeders, but I didn't know the name of the condition until I was diagnosed in the 1970s. We have type 2A VWD.

VWD has had a profound effect on our family. My father's father bled to death from an ulcer when he was 27. His widow did not believe she could raise their three children, Ernest, age 7, Richard, age 5, and Dorothy, age 3, alone. She put them in an orphanage in Greensboro, North Carolina, not far from where they had lived. Dorothy, my aunt, was sent to a Catholic convent and raised by the nuns there. Ernest, my father, and Richard, my uncle, were taken in by a family in Drewry, North Carolina, where they were treated like slaves. When my father was 16, he and his brother, Richard, along with another boy the family had taken in, ran away. My father didn't see his mother again until he was in his thirties.

My bleeding problems began when I was 18 months old. I knocked out my lower four teeth and my gums wouldn't stop bleeding. Finally, a cup of ice and tea bags brought the bleeding under control. Later, I fell and bit my tongue. Again, the bleeding was very hard to control. Once I had my fingers crushed by a jack. The blood in the sink was two inches deep. My whole life, I have suffered from nosebleeds.

My mother was afraid that if I were drafted and sent to Vietnam, I would get injured and bleed to death. She insisted that I see a specialist. That's when I was diagnosed with von Willebrand disease.

The first time I ever received any prophylaxis to prevent bleeding was when I had my wisdom teeth removed at the age of 26. I was admitted to the hospital before the surgery and received clotting factor VIII and cryoprecipitate. I still bled during the surgery. I received cryoprecipitate every day for one to two weeks afterward, but I continued to have bleeding complications. I was out of work for a month and a half.

I was in a car wreck on Interstate 95 in 1979, but after my experience having my wisdom teeth out, I was afraid to go to the hospital. Fortunately, I didn't have any bleeding problems, but I did have neck and back pain. I wound up having an EMG. (An EMG is an electromyogram, a test for nerve damage, which uses needles that are inserted into the muscles.) Although I didn't have any bleeding after the car wreck, I did have bleeding from those needles!

I was the youngest of six children. Two of my sisters also have von Willebrand disease. They have both suffered serious bleeding problems and have ports (indwelling intravenous catheters) because of their frequent need for prophylaxis (with clotting factor concentrates). My daughter is also affected. She just gave birth to her first child without problems, but she required daily infusions of [a VWF/FVIII concentrate] for three weeks afterward.

11. What is the difference between VWD and hemophilia?

Von Willebrand disease results from insufficient, abnormal, or absent von Willebrand factor. Because VWF is especially important for the prevention of bleeding from skin and mucous membranes (the lining of the nose, mouth, intestines, uterus, and vagina), bleeding is common at these sites. Hemophilia results from a deficiency of clotting factor VIII (hemophilia A) or clotting factor IX (hemophilia B). Because factors VIII and IX are especially important for the prevention of bleeding within deep tissues, bleeding is common in joints and within muscles.

While VWD is generally inherited by autosomal dominant transmission (see Question 10), hemophilia is generally inherited by sex-linked or X-linked transmission. An X-linked genetic disease is one that is generally passed on from a mother to her son. Humans have 23 pairs of chromosomes of which one pair is the sex chromosomes. Females have two X chromosomes. Males have one X chromosome and one Y chromosome. Males inherit a Y chromosome from their fathers and an X chromosome from their mothers. Abnormal genes on the X chromosome from the mother will result in a 50% chance of her having an affected son. The mother herself, who has a second normal X chromosome, is not affected or only mildly affected. She is generally referred to as a carrier. Since the genes for clotting factors VIII and IX are located on the X chromosome, an abnormal gene for either factor VIII or factor IX will result in hemophilia in the affected male. In order for a female to be affected, she would need to have an abnormal gene on both of her X chromosomes, or have one X chromosome with an abnormal gene and a second X chromosome that was inactive or nonexistent. Consequently, hemophilia very rarely affects girls or women.

Hemophilia very rarely affects girls or women.

Hemophilia is usually severe and requires frequent infusions of clotting factor concentrates (more than once a week) to control or prevent bleeding. Von Willebrand disease is usually mild or moderate and rarely requires infusions of clotting factor concentrates to control or prevent bleeding except prior to surgery or procedures.

Hemophilia is relatively rare, affecting about 1 in 5,000 males. Von Willebrand disease is more common.

12. How common is VWD?

In general, mild disease is common and severe disease is rare. Based on studies of individuals with bleeding symptoms, a family history of bleeding, and low levels of von Willebrand factor, VWD affects as many as 1 in 100 individuals. Experts who treat VWD, however, question whether it is this common. Based on the numbers of individuals enrolled at **hemophilia treatment centers**, VWD affects only 1 in 10,000 individuals. Nonetheless, there are probably many people with mild VWD who have never been diagnosed. Type 1 disease may affect as many as 1 in 100 individuals, type 2 disease is uncommon, and type 3 disease is rare, affecting as few as 1 in 250,000 to 1 in 1,000,000 individuals.

A family history of a bleeding disorder provides an important clue.

13. How is VWD diagnosed?

Von Willebrand disease is sometimes difficult to diagnose. Many people with the condition do not have serious bleeding and do not get diagnosed until they have an episode of heavy bleeding. The diagnosis is made based on the presence of symptoms and the results of certain laboratory tests. A family history of a bleeding disorder provides an important clue. Since there are several types of VWD, and because existing laboratory tests have limitations, no single laboratory test can diagnose the condition. When a bleeding disorder is suspected, the initial laboratory tests should include a **complete blood count (CBC)** and tests to make sure there is no clotting factor deficiency. These tests include a **prothrombin time (PT)**, **activated partial thromboplastin time (aPTT)**, and fibrinogen level (or thrombin clot time). While these tests may be useful for making sure that there is no clotting factor deficiency, even the aPTT may be normal in patients with VWD (see Questions 14, 15, and 16).

The next series of tests includes specific tests for VWD including **von Willebrand ristocetin cofactor activity (VWF:RCo), von Willebrand factor antigen (VWF:Ag)**, and factor VIII (FVIII). The results of these tests may vary depending on a person's age, race, other genetic factors, blood type, stress, inflammation, and hormones. Other

Hemophilia treatment center (HTC)

A clinic where a team of doctors, nurses, social workers, physical therapists, and other specialists work together to deliver comprehensive, state-of-the-art care to people with bleeding disorders.

Complete blood count (CBC)

A test for determining if anemia is present and how severe the anemia is, and for determining if thrombocytopenia (an insufficient number of platelets) is present.

Prothrombin time (PT)

A blood test that measures the length of time (in seconds) that it takes for clotting to occur when tissue factor and other substances are added to the liquid portion of blood in a test tube.

Activated partial thromboplastin time (aPTT)

A blood test that measures the length of time (in seconds) that it takes for clotting to occur when certain substances are added to the plasma or liquid portion of blood in a test tube.

von Willebrand ristocetin cofactor activity (VWF:RCo)

A test that measures the function of von Willebrand factor (VWF).

von Willebrand factor antigen (VWF:Ag)

A test that measures the actual amount of von Willebrand factor (VWF) protein in a patient's plasma.

PFA-100®

An automated test of platelet function.

Hematologist

A doctor who is a specialist in the field of medicine that involves the study and treatment of blood disorders.

factors that can affect the results of these tests are how the sample is processed and the quality of the laboratory. Often, tests must be repeated several times over several months. In many instances, only one of these specific tests may be abnormal. Further testing to determine the type of VWD includes assessment of von Willebrand multimers, among other studies.

Screening tests are simple, inexpensive tests that can suggest whether a disease is present. The bleeding time, which has been suggested as a screening test for VWD, requires a small cut, is painful, produces variable results, does not detect all cases of VWD, and when it is abnormal, may not be abnormal due to VWD. Recently, several automated tests of platelet function have been developed. One of the tests, the **PFA-100®**, has been found to detect a high percentage of cases of VWD, but by the time an individual is suspected of having VWD and is referred to a **hematologist**, the hematologist will want to make a definitive diagnosis and will not want to miss a case of VWD. Therefore, he or she will order a panel of tests for VWD, which are mentioned above and described below.

14. What is a complete blood count?

A complete blood count (CBC) is a blood test that measures:

1. The amount of hemoglobin in the blood
2. The fraction of blood that is composed of red blood cells (the hematocrit)
3. The number of platelets
4. The number of white blood cells
5. The size of the red blood cells or mean corpuscular volume (MCV)

6. The amount of hemoglobin within the red blood cells or mean corpuscular hemoglobin (MCH)

7. The concentration of hemoglobin within the red blood cells or mean corpuscular hemoglobin concentration (MCHC)

A complete blood count is useful for determining if anemia is present and how severe the anemia is. It is also useful for determining if thrombocytopenia (an insufficient number of platelets) is present. Thrombocytopenia can also result in bleeding.

A complete blood count is useful for determining if anemia is present and how severe the anemia is.

15. What is the activated partial thromboplastin time test?

The activated partial thromboplastin time (aPTT) test is a blood test that measures the length of time (in seconds) that it takes for clotting to occur when certain substances are added to the plasma or liquid portion of blood in a test tube. A normal result requires normal levels of clotting factors VIII, IX, XI, and XII; normal levels of pre-kallikrein and high-molecular-weight kininogen, as well as normal levels of factors V, X, prothrombin, and fibrinogen. If the prothrombin time (PT) test is normal, the aPTT can be used to detect deficiencies of clotting factors VIII, IX, XI, and XII. If the factor VIII level is low in an individual with VWD, the aPTT test may be abnormal, but if the factor VIII level is 50% of normal or more, the aPTT will likely be normal. For this reason, the aPTT cannot be relied on to detect VWD. If the aPTT is prolonged and the factor VIII level is normal, another factor deficiency, particularly deficiency of factor XI, should be suspected.

16. What is the prothrombin time test?

The prothrombin time (PT) test is a blood test that measures the length of time (in seconds) that it takes for clotting to occur when tissue factor and other substances are added to the liquid portion of blood in a test tube. A normal result requires normal levels of clotting factor VII, as well as normal levels of factors V, X, prothrombin, and fibrinogen. If the activated partial thromboplastin time (aPTT) test is normal, the PT can be used to detect deficiencies of factor VII. The PT should be normal in individuals with VWD.

17. What is the von Willebrand ristocetin cofactor activity test?

The von Willebrand ristocetin cofactor activity (VWF: RCo) test measures the function of von Willebrand factor. Specifically, the test measures the ability of a patient's VWF to interact with normal platelets. The test uses ristocetin, an antibiotic that was never marketed because it caused platelets to clump or aggregate and resulted in thrombocytopenia. The VWF:RCo test capitalizes on ristocetin's ability to aggregate platelets. There are different methods of performing the test, but all look for platelet clumping or aggregation after adding a patient's plasma to normal platelets. If a patient has low levels of VWF, abnormal VWF, or absent VWF, the platelets will not clump or aggregate normally. Varying dilutions of the patient's plasma are used to estimate the degree of VWF activity present. Results are reported in international units per deciliter (IU/dL) based on World Health Organization (WHO) standards.

18. What is the von Willebrand factor antigen test?

The von Willebrand factor antigen (VWF:Ag) test measures the actual amount of VWF protein in a patient's plasma, but does not give information about the functionality of the VWF that is present. Results are reported in international units per deciliter (IU/dL). The VWF:Ag value does not provide information about the qualitative hemostatic function or activity of VWF; for example, these tests can be normal in patients with type 2 VWD.

19. What is the factor VIII test?

The factor VIII (FVIII) test is usually performed by measuring the ability of a patient's plasma to shorten the time it takes factor VIII–deficient plasma to clot. Results are reported in international units per deciliter (IU/dL).

20. What is the test for von Willebrand factor multimers?

A more specialized test is used to evaluate the presence and size of von Willebrand factor multimers. Von Willebrand factor multimers are identified in a patient's plasma using an antibody. Various methods are used to depict the variable concentrations of different-sized multimers.

21. Are there genetic tests for von Willebrand disease?

There are tests that can be used to look for mutations in the von Willebrand factor gene. These mutations are much more likely to be present in the more severe forms of VWD and less likely to be present in the milder forms of the disease, where other factors, such as blood type, may play a role. At the moment, these genetic tests are performed only in certain research centers and are not available at other coagulation laboratories.

22. Where can I go to get tested for von Willebrand disease?

A good place to start is by visiting your family physician.

A good place to start is by visiting your family physician. A family practitioner, internist, obstetrician gynecologist, or pediatrician should be able to refer you to a hematologist or hemophilia treatment center for testing. Not all laboratories have the capability of performing tests for von Willebrand disease, so you might have to travel some distance to get tested.

23. Who should be tested for von Willebrand disease?

Individuals with unexplained bleeding symptoms should be evaluated for a bleeding disorder.

The following are specific signs and symptoms of VWD:

- Prolonged bleeding from trivial wounds, lasting more than 15 minutes or recurring spontaneously during the 7 days after the wound
- Heavy, prolonged, or recurrent bleeding after surgery such as a tonsillectomy
- Bruising with minimal or no trauma, especially bruising resulting in a lump
- Nosebleeds that last more than 10 minutes or require medical attention to stop

- Heavy, prolonged, or recurrent bleeding after dental procedures or tooth extraction
- Unexplained bleeding from the stomach or intestines
- Anemia requiring iron therapy or transfusion
- Heavy menstrual bleeding requiring more than one pad or tampon in an hour's time or resulting in clots an inch or more in diameter

24. Are there other conditions that resemble VWD?

Several other conditions resemble VWD. While the bleeding patterns for these conditions may be different, factor deficiencies including factor XI deficiency and deficiency of factor VIII (hemophilia A or hemophilia A carrier status) or factor IX (hemophilia B or hemophilia B carrier status) may resemble VWD. Platelet disorders can also resemble VWD. In fact, platelet disorders may be as common as VWD and may have very similar symptoms. As discussed in Question 3, when blood vessels are injured and the endothelium and the tissue underneath it are damaged, the subendothelium is exposed. The subendothelium is composed of the protein collagen, which is rough and sticky. Platelets, the cells that prevent blood from leaking out of an injured blood vessel, stick or adhere to the subendothelium where it is exposed. Abnormalities not only of platelets but also of collagen, such as occur with a condition known as Ehlers–Danlos syndrome, can result in bleeding tendencies similar to those that occur with VWD.

People who take anticoagulant medication or antiplatelet medication for a history of deep vein thrombosis, pulmonary embolism, heart attack, or stroke may have symptoms similar to those of people with VWD.

25. Should my family members be tested for VWD?

Since your parents, brothers, sisters, and children may also have VWD, you should inform them about a diagnosis of VWD in the family. If your children have symptoms, inform their physician and have them tested. Other adult family members may want more information about the likelihood of having VWD and the consequences of the diagnosis before they are tested. Ideally, they should have the opportunity to meet with a knowledgeable genetic counselor before they are tested.

With the right treatment, people who have VWD can lead normal, active lives and expect to live as long as anyone else.

26. What is the life expectancy of people with von Willebrand disease?

Von Willebrand disease cannot be cured, but it can be treated. With the right treatment, people who have VWD can lead normal, active lives and expect to live as long as anyone else.

PART TWO

Treatment

How is von Willebrand factor replaced?

What are topical agents and how can they help?

What if I have to have an operation or other procedure? How is bleeding prevented?

More . . .

27. How is VWD treated?

The treatment of VWD depends on the type of VWD and how severe it is. Most cases of VWD are mild and may only require treatment at the time of surgery, dental procedures, or injury. When treatment is required, bleeding symptoms are controlled where they occur, by using medications to reduce the risk of bleeding and by raising von Willebrand factor. There are two strategies for raising VWF. One is to administer **DDAVP**, which causes VWF to be released from the endothelial cells that line blood vessels. The other is to administer human plasma–derived, virally inactivated clotting factor concentrates.

DDAVP

Also known as desmopressin, DDAVP is a synthetic version of the hormone vasopressin, which raises von Willebrand factor (VWF) levels by causing VWF to be released from the endothelial cells that line blood vessels.

28. What is DDAVP?

DDAVP, which is also known as desmopressin, is a synthetic version of the hormone vasopressin and has been used to treat VWD for more than 25 years. DDAVP is an abbreviation for 1-deamino-8-D-arginine vasopressin. DDAVP raises von Willebrand factor levels by causing VWF to be released from the Weibel-Palade bodies, where it is stored in the endothelial cells that line blood vessels. In patients who respond to DDAVP, DDAVP can raise VWF levels two- to fivefold. DDAVP, however, can raise VWF levels only if VWF is present in the Weibel-Palade bodies. Most patients with type 1 VWD and some patients with type 2A and type 2M VWD respond to DDAVP, but patients with type 3 VWD do not. DDAVP also raises factor VIII levels, but the reason is unknown.

Vicki's story (type 3 VWD):

In 1985, my doctor admitted me to the hospital for a bleed in my elbow, again at a military hospital. He knew about factor VIII concentrates and said they would not work for me, but he had heard of a new drug called DDAVP that was working for VWD and might be a possibility. While I was in the hospital, he "challenged" me with a DDAVP infusion (see Question 31) We were so hopeful. The doctor sat beside me for the whole test and administered the infusion himself, but nothing happened. As a result, I had to continue as I had with no real treatment. He also tested me for HIV. What a stressful two-week waiting period that was!!

Jessica's story (type 1 VWD):

My body responds very well to the DDAVP, and after trying a few different pharmaceutical options to control my bleeding, I have decided to stick with this. I use it primarily when I get a bloody nose, but also when I have a heavy period. My hematologist also recommended that I take a dose before I got my (small) tattoo.

29. What are the side effects of DDAVP?

Minor side effects of DDAVP are common. DDAVP can cause flushing of the face, changes in blood pressure, headaches, and stomach or intestinal upsets. These are unpleasant side effects but are not reasons to discontinue the medication. A serious side effect of DDAVP, however, is a low concentration of sodium in the blood. Because DDAVP is a synthetic version of the hormone vasopressin, an "antidiuretic" hormone, it can cause water to be retained, diluting the blood and lowering the concentration of sodium, an essential mineral. A single dose of DDAVP in a healthy adult is unlikely to cause a problem, but if repeated doses are necessary, fluids should be restricted for 24 hours. Otherwise, a dangerously low concentration of sodium could result in seizures. Because this is more likely to occur in young children, most pediatric hematologists do not prescribe DDAVP to children under the age of 2.

DDAVP can cause flushing of the face, changes in blood pressure, headaches, and stomach or intestinal upsets.

Of course, DDAVP raises VWF levels and increases the tendency of blood to clot. In theory, this could increase the risk of a blood **clot**, including a heart attack or stroke. In fact, there have been cases of heart attack occurring after individuals took DDAVP. For this reason DDAVP is used with caution, if at all, in individuals who are elderly or have risk factors for heart attack and stroke.

Andra's story (low VWF or mild type 1 VWD):

In 1998, I had a cheilectomy, surgery for arthritis in the joint between my left big toe and my foot. I had the surgery before I was diagnosed with von Willebrand disease or low von Willebrand factor. Prior to the surgery, I am sure that I was asked if I had ever had any bleeding problems and I am sure that I would have said no. I regarded my heavy menstrual bleeding as normal and my only previous surgery, for impacted wisdom teeth, did not require a transfusion. Although my face had turned purple and swelled to the point that I was unrecognizable afterward, I did not think that that was abnormal. The evening after the cheilectomy, the pain was minimal and I shunned the Percocet® in favor of Motrin®, a nonsteroidal anti-inflammatory drug [see Question 86]. That night, I bled through the dressing on my foot. I paged the resident physician, but got no response, so I peeled the soggy dressing off and examined my foot. It was swollen to what appeared to be almost twice normal size, it was purple, and it was oozing. I wrapped it well in some gauze I had at home and the oozing subsided. It took two months before I could get it into a normal shoe.

In 2003, I had the same procedure on the opposite foot. This time, I was pretreated with DDAVP. I can't say I liked the way the DDAVP made me feel. I became flushed and woozy. It made me nauseous and gave me a headache, but within a very short time I went to sleep for my surgery and woke up feeling fine. Any side effects from the DDAVP were worth it.

Besides receiving the DDAVP, I refrained from taking any nonsteroidal anti-inflammatory drugs. After the surgery, I did not bleed through the dressing. My foot did not ooze, turn purple, or swell. I was back in a normal shoe within three weeks. What a difference the DDAVP made!

30. How is DDAVP administered?

DDAVP can be inhaled through the nose (nasal administration), injected under the skin (subcutaneous administration), or infused into a vein (intravenous administration). Nasal administration requires high-dose DDAVP (Stimate®) and is effective in preventing minor bleeding. Intravenous administration of DDAVP is required to prevent major bleeding. Two studies found that the dose of DDAVP that resulted in the highest level of factor VIII in the blood was 0.3 micrograms per kilogram and the highest level of von Willebrand factor was 0.2 to 0.3 micrograms per kilogram of body weight. (A kilogram is equal to 2.2 pounds.) Therefore, the dose of DDAVP that is used when given intravenously is 0.3 micrograms per kilogram of body weight. The dose for subcutaneous administration is the same as the dose for intravenous administration, but the subcutaneous formulation of DDAVP is not available in the United States. The dose for nasal administration is two puffs (one to each nostril) of a solution containing 150 micrograms per puff. The dose is only one puff (to a single nostril) for an individual weighing less than 50 kilograms (110 pounds).

Because DDAVP raises VWF levels by causing VWF to be released from the Weibel-Palade bodies, not by causing more VWF to be formed, repeated doses are less and less effective. For this reason, and because DDAVP can cause a low concentration of sodium in the blood, doses should not be repeated more frequently than every 24 hours or for more than two to three days in a row.

31. What is a trial of DDAVP or DDAVP challenge test?

A trial of DDAVP is the administration of DDAVP solely for the purpose of seeing how an individual will respond to it. A trial of DDAVP is most likely to be performed in individuals with ristocetin cofactor activity levels between 10 and 20 IU/dL. Individuals with levels below 10 IU/dL are less likely to have an adequate response. When performed with intravenous DDAVP, the standard dose of 0.3 micrograms per kilogram of body weight is used. The von Willebrand ristocetin cofactor activity (VWF:RCo) is measured 30 to 60 minutes after DDAVP administration. A doubling or tripling of VWF:RCo, or a level of at least 30 IU/dL, is considered a successful response. A successful response with intravenous administration does not guarantee a successful response with nasal administration, so prior to relying on Stimate® to prevent bleeding, an individual may undergo another trial with nasal administration of DDAVP.

32. How is von Willebrand factor replaced?

von Willebrand factor concentrate

A product purified from human plasma that is rich in von Willebrand factor.

Von Willebrand factor is replaced with clotting factor products, specifically **von Willebrand factor concentrates**, derived from purified human plasma. Most of these products were developed up to 20 years ago as factor VIII concentrates to treat hemophilia A. The significant amount of VWF in some of these products led them to being used to treat VWD. Therefore, these

VWF concentrates contain not only VWF, but factor VIII, fibrinogen, and other plasma proteins that have been dried and purified. During the purification process, viruses are inactivated, including potentially harmful viruses. Although the remote risk of virus transmission exists, because of improved selection of plasma donors, testing of donated plasma, and improved virus inactivation processes, no transmission of human immunodeficiency virus (HIV), hepatitis B, or hepatitis C has occurred with any VWF concentrates currently marketed in the United States.

Blood products, such as **fresh frozen plasma** and cryoprecipitate, are tested for known viruses but are not purified, and thus may allow unknown but potentially harmful viruses to be transmitted.

Fresh frozen plasma (FFP)

Plasma frozen shortly after being obtained from donors to preserve the clotting factors.

Reconstituted VWF concentrates are administered intravenously (infused into a vein). They are used by patients with VWD who do not respond to DDAVP or by patients with VWD who are experiencing a major bleeding episode, undergoing major surgery, or giving birth and thus require an extended duration of therapy.

Vicki's story (type 3 VWD):

At age 40, I needed my first surgery, which was to remove my wisdom teeth. Yikes, I had been through this two times before: no one would take me into surgery, no one could get my bleeding time into normal range. I must have given the hemophilia treatment center (HTC) nurse the weirdest look. . . . I know I said nooooooo, I am going to die with these wisdom teeth as all surgeries before had been cancelled. The nurse calmly looked at me and said that factor replacement concentrates would be given to me prior to surgery and that would bring me into normal bleeding ranges. Again with disbelief, but a trust in the medical system, I said okay and scheduled the procedure. I talked with my husband and parents about taking care of the kids, fully expecting to be in the hospital for at least a week and then needing to recuperate at home for another week. My parents moved in for the duration and I proceeded to the hospital.

I was admitted through the same day surgical unit and waited for the HTC nurse to arrive. All this time the other nurses were prepping me for surgery and I was getting more nervous. The HTC nurse arrived and asked me if I was ready. I said I was not ready until I had received the factor infusion and then looked at the factor VIII activity level results. Low and behold, the factor VIII results came back at 150% (mine were usually less than 12%). I was wheeled into the operating room and the next I knew, I was waking up convinced that the procedure had been cancelled and I needed to go home. I felt discomfort in one jaw and asked the nurse if they were only able to get one tooth out. She said no they took all four and it went very well. Okay, now I just had to get through the residual bleeding and swelling that I had heard about from friends and family. The hematologist came in and looked at me and told me that she and the surgeon considered this a bloodless procedure from the small amount of bleeding that occurred. I was settled into the room where I expected to be for the next week and spent the night with cold compresses on my face as well as another transfusion of factor replacement concentrate. The next morning, after another dose of factor, the HTC nurse told me that I could go home!! Imagine, only one night in the hospital! I had limited swelling and no bruising. Imagine my mother's surprise when I walked into the house later that day! She asked what was wrong, what had happened, I told her that I was okay; I had the teeth to prove they had been pulled and all I needed was additional factor infusions for the next week. The whole family was amazed at what factor had done for this situation. Why didn't I know about this stuff the year before when my shoulder went out and hurt like the dickens for six weeks straight? I did not even realize that I was bleeding; I considered it arthritis.

This was the start of my love affair with factor replacement concentrates. I was 40 years old and finally had something to control my bleeding. I learned that I could use factor as bleeds occur and not just in life-and-death situations as I had been told six years earlier. I also found out that concentrates for VWD had been around since 1985. I was astounded!!

33. What are the side effects of factor replacement?

The most serious side effect of factor replacement is allergic reactions. These reactions can include hives, rashes, itching, swelling, and, more ominously, difficulty breathing and a drop in blood pressure. Allergic reactions require discontinuation of the infusion and immediate treatment to counteract the symptoms. The purer the product the less likely an allergic reaction will occur. For instance, allergic reactions are less likely to occur with VWF concentrates than with fresh frozen plasma or cryoprecipitate (see Questions 45 and 46). A rare side effect of factor replacement is blood clots. Blood clots are more likely to occur in individuals with risk factors and are less likely to occur if, during replacement, the von Willebrand ristocetin cofactor activity (VWF:RCo) is not allowed to rise to more than 200 IU/dL and the factor VIII level is not allowed to rise to more than 250 to 300 IU/dL.

Allergic reactions require discontinuation of the infusion and immediate treatment to counteract the symptoms.

34. What is Humate-P®?

Humate-P® (known as Hemate-P® in Europe) was originally developed more than 20 years ago to treat hemophilia A and, in 1999, became the first plasma-derived clotting factor product approved by the United States Food and Drug Administration (FDA) to treat VWD. The FDA recently approved Humate-P® to prevent bleeding at the time of surgery in patients with VWD. Humate-P® contains about twice as much VWF as factor VIII. Humate-P® is marketed in the United States by the CSL Behring Company.

35. What is Alphanate®?

Alphanate® is another plasma-derived clotting factor product used to treat hemophilia A. The FDA recently approved Alphanate® to prevent bleeding at the time of surgery in patients with type 1 and type 2 VWD. Alphanate® contains between half and equal amounts of VWF as factor VIII. Alphanate® is manufactured by Grifols Biologicals, Inc.

36. What is Koāte®?

Koāte® is another plasma-derived clotting factor product used to treat hemophilia A. The FDA has not yet approved Koāte® to treat patients with VWD. Koāte® contains less than half as much VWF as factor VIII. Koāte® is manufactured by Talecris Biotherapeutics.

During the past years, two VWF concentrates have been developed specifically for the treatment of VWD.

37. What is Wilfactin?

During the past years, two VWF concentrates have been developed specifically for the treatment of VWD. The first one, Wilfactin®, is a byproduct of factor VIII manufacturing and thus contains only small amounts of active factor VIII. Minimal factor VIII is not necessarily desirable, since many individuals with von Willebrand factor also have low factor VIII levels and need adequate factor VIII levels for normal blood clotting. Wilfactin®, which is not available in the United States, is manufactured by LLB Therapeutics (France).

38. What is Wilate®?

Wilate® is the second of two VWF concentrates that have been developed specifically for the treatment of VWD. It is comprised of almost equal amounts of active VWF and factor VIII. Wilate® is manufactured by Octapharma in Austria from United States plasma. It is available in many countries worldwide, but at the time of publication, it was not yet available in the United States.

39. What is Amicar®?

Amicar®, or ε-aminocaproic acid, is an **antifibrinolytic** medication, a medication that can reduce the risk of bleeding. Antifibrinolytic medications help prevent normal blood clots that have formed at the site of blood vessel injury from being broken down or lysed. Fibrin forms the mesh or net that holds platelets firmly in place in a stable blood clot. Antifibrinolytic medications bind to plasminogen, the enzyme or specialized protein that breaks down fibrin and prevent plasminogen from breaking down blood clots. Amicar® can be taken by mouth or administered intravenously (infused into a vein). Amicar® can be used to prevent and control bleeding at the time of surgery, injury, menstruation, or childbirth. Because the lining of the mouth is rich in plasminogen, Amicar® is thought to be especially effective in preventing bleeding at the time of dental or other oral surgery. Side effects of Amicar® include nausea, vomiting, diarrhea, abdominal pain, and

Antifibrinolytic

A medication that can reduce the risk of bleeding by preventing normal blood clots that have formed at the site of blood vessel injury from being broken down or lysed.

muscle cramps. In theory, Amicar® could increase the risk of abnormal blood clots.

Garry's story (type 2A VWD):

I moved to North Carolina in 1999. In 2000 I had dental surgery and received DDAVP. My sister told me about Amicar®. I have had some dental procedures since then without DDAVP, but have taken a lot of Amicar®. I take ten pills every six hours. I'm nauseated, but I don't bleed. In 2004, I had some teeth pulled. I didn't even tell the dentist about my VWD. If they know you have VWD, they don't want to touch you. I took lots of Amicar® and didn't have a problem.

40. What is tranexamic acid?

Tranexamic acid, or Cyklokapron®, is another antifibrinolytic medication, a medication that can reduce the risk of bleeding (see Question 34). It, too, binds to plasminogen, the enzyme that breaks down fibrin, and prevents plasminogen from breaking down blood clots. Like Amicar®, tranexamic acid can be taken by mouth or administered intravenously (infused into a vein). Tranexamic acid can also be used to prevent and control bleeding at the time of surgery, injury, menstruation, or childbirth. Tranexamic acid seems to have fewer stomach and intestinal side effects than Amicar®. A rare side effect of tranexamic acid is changes in color vision. Changes in color vision require discontinuation of the medication and evaluation by an ophthalmologist. In theory, tranexamic could also increase the risk of abnormal blood clots, but studies have not shown this to be true.

Tranexamic acid can also be used to prevent and control bleeding at the time of surgery, injury, menstruation, or childbirth.

41. What are topical agents and how can they help?

Topical agents are medications that can be applied directly to tissue to stop bleeding. They can be used to stop oozing from small, sometimes inaccessible, capillaries or small venules during surgery (see Question 2). One of these agents is FloSeal™. The active ingredient in FloSeal™ is a thrombin component derived from human plasma. Thrombin is the active version of prothrombin or clotting factor II, an enzyme or specialized protein that converts fibrinogen to fibrin (see Question 3). Thrombin-JMI® is another topical agent. The active ingredient is bovine thrombin, thrombin derived from cows or cattle. A problem with bovine thrombin is the possibility of the development of antibodies (specialized proteins) that can interfere with a person's own thrombin. Products with bovine thrombin are, therefore, less likely to be used. TISSEEL is another topical agent. TISSEEL is referred to as a fibrin sealant or fibrin glue. There are three active ingredients in TISSEEL. They are thrombin, derived from human plasma; fibrinogen, also derived from human plasma; and aprotinin, an inhibitor of clot breakdown or fibrinolysis, that comes from cows or cattle. When mixed together, the thrombin and fibrinogen form a clot. The aprotinin prevents the clot from breaking down.

In theory, topical agents derived from human plasma could transmit viruses, but during the purification process, viruses are inactivated, including potentially harmful viruses. Because of improved selection of plasma donors, testing of donated plasma, and improved virus inactivation processes, the risk of virus transmission is very, very small.

Topical agents
Medications that can be applied directly to tissue to stop bleeding.

Because of improved selection of plasma donors, testing of donated plasma, and improved virus inactivation processes, the risk of virus transmission is very, very small.

There are other topical agents that have not necessarily been tried in patients with VWD but could be used to control bleeding. BioGlue® is an animal-based sealant that is made of a bovine serum albumin (a cow protein) and a chemical called glutaraldehyde. The cow protein and the chemical join with a patient's tissue to seal the area, like with a glue. BioGlue® is used to help seal leaks around sutures (surgical stitches) or staples in large blood vessels at the time of surgery involving these vessels. Another of these topical agents is CoSeal®, which is used to help prevent leaking at the site of blood vessel repair. It is made from polyethylene glycol and does not contain any human or animal protein. Another one of these topical agents is QuikClot®, a granular product made from zeolite, a very porous natural mineral. QuikClot® can be poured directly into wounds. It stops bleeding by absorbing water from blood, concentrating clotting factors, and activating platelets. It is carried by armed forces medical personnel for use in treating battle wounds but can also be purchased in drug stores for use by civilians.

42. What is fresh frozen plasma?

Plasma is obtained by separating the liquid portion of blood from the cells. Fresh frozen plasma (FFP) is frozen shortly after being obtained from donors to preserve the clotting factors. It can be stored up to one year and thawed just before use. It is transfused in cases of multiple clotting factor deficiencies.

43. What are the risks of fresh frozen plasma?

Although plasma donors are screened for infections and the plasma collected from donors is tested for known viruses, fresh frozen plasma does not undergo a purification process like clotting factor concentrates do. There is a risk that unknown viruses will be transmitted. The risk of transmission of known viruses from a single unit is very small (1 in 1,000,000 for HIV and 1 in 900,000 for hepatitis C), but the risk exists.

44. What is cryoprecipitate?

Cryoprecipitate is created from plasma by freezing it, slowly thawing it, then finally centrifuging it (a process that separates it by spinning it at very high speeds). The lower portion, the precipitate, is rich in clotting factors, including factor VIII, fibrinogen, and von Willebrand factor. While cryoprecipitate contains VWF, it is not recommended except in emergency situations when VWF concentrates are not available.

Cryoprecipitate
A product rich in factor VIII, fibrinogen, and von Willebrand factor (VWF) that is created from plasma by freezing it, slowly thawing it, then finally centrifuging it (a process that separates it by spinning it at very high speeds).

45. What are the risks of cryoprecipitate?

Although plasma donors are screened for infections and the plasma used to create cryoprecipitate is tested for known viruses, cryoprecipitate does not undergo a purification process. As is true with fresh frozen plasma (FFP), there is a risk that unknown viruses will be transmitted. The risk of transmission of known viruses from a single unit is very small (1 in 1,000,000 for HIV and 1 in 900,000 for hepatitis C), but the risk exists.

46. Does an ordinary blood transfusion have von Willebrand factor in it?

Blood may be transfused as whole blood or as one of its components. Up to four components may be derived from one unit of blood. These include platelets, plasma, cryoprecipitate, and red blood cells. Since most patients seldom require all of the components of whole blood, it makes sense to transfuse only that portion of blood needed by the patient for a specific condition or disease. This treatment, referred to as blood component therapy, allows several patients to benefit from one unit of donated whole blood. Therefore, whole blood is rarely available and rarely transfused. While whole blood does contain VWF, an ordinary blood transfusion of red blood cells, from which the plasma has been removed, does not.

Whole blood is rarely available and rarely transfused.

47. What if I have to have an operation or other procedure? How is bleeding prevented?

How bleeding is prevented depends on the bleeding tendency of the individual and the bleeding risk of the surgery. Prior to minor surgery, von Willebrand ristocetin cofactor activity (VWF:RCo) and factor VIII levels should be at least 30 IU/dL and preferably higher than 50 IU/dL. These levels should be maintained for at least one to five days. These levels may be achieved with DDAVP or may require factor replacement with von Willebrand factor concentrates. For individuals with mild or moderate von Willebrand disease undergoing oral surgery, antifibrinolytics (Amicar® or tranexamic acid) and/or topical agents such as fibrin sealant and bovine thrombin may be used along with DDAVP or VWF concentrates to prevent bleeding.

If you are undergoing major surgery you should insist on having your operation at a medical center with a hemophilia treatment center or similar hemostasis center. This center should have a laboratory capable of performing specialized coagulation tests 24 hours a day, a pharmacy with VWF concentrates, and a knowledgeable hematologist, surgeon, and anesthesiologist. Prior to major surgery, your VWF:RCo and factor VIII levels should be at least 100 IU/dL. These levels should be maintained for at least 7 to 14 days. Adequate factor levels are necessary not only to prevent bleeding but to promote normal wound healing. These levels will usually require factor replacement with VWF concentrates. Close monitoring is required to prevent levels from dropping below 50 IU/dL, which would increase the risk of bleeding, or from rising above 200 to 300 IU/dL (VWF:RCo greater than 200 IU/dL and factor VIII greater than 250–300 IU/dL), which would increase the risk of abnormal blood clots.

48. What if I am injured? How will the bleeding be stopped?

How the bleeding will be stopped will depend on the nature of your injury and on your bleeding tendency. Besides employing all the usual emergency procedures that are necessary to stop bleeding, doctors will want to ensure that a patient with VWD has adequate von Willebrand ristocetin cofactor activity (VWF:RCo) and factor VIII levels. Adequate levels are necessary not only to control bleeding but to promote normal wound healing.

After a minor injury, your VWF:RCo and factor VIII levels should be at least 30 IU/dL, preferably 50 IU/dL, and maintained at these levels for at least one to five days. These levels may be achieved with DDAVP or may require factor replacement with VWF concentrates. Antifibrinolytics (Amicar® or tranexamic acid) and/or topical agents such as fibrin sealant and bovine thrombin may be used along with DDAVP or VWF concentrates to stop bleeding.

If you have major bleeding, your VWF:RCo and factor VIII levels should be at least 100 IU/dL. These levels should be maintained for at least 7 to 14 days. These levels will usually require factor replacement with VWF concentrates. In an emergency situation, if VWF concentrates are unavailable, cryoprecipitate may be substituted. Continued major bleeding, however, should be treated at a medical center with a hemophilia treatment center or similar hemostasis center where VWF concentrates are available. This center should have not only a pharmacy with VWF concentrates but also a laboratory capable of performing specialized coagulation tests 24 hours a day and a knowledgeable hematologist, surgeon, and anesthesiologist. Like after major surgery, close monitoring is required to prevent factor levels from dropping below 50 IU/dL, which would increase the risk of bleeding, or from rising above 200 to 300 IU/dL, which would increase the risk of abnormal blood clots.

49. Can a person with VWD still have a blood clot (deep vein thrombosis, pulmonary embolism, heart attack, or stroke)?

Yes, unfortunately, a person with VWD or other bleeding disorder can still have a blood clot, especially if he or she has other risk factors. Blood clotting factors play an important role in the development of deep vein thrombosis and pulmonary embolism (the consequence of a deep vein thrombosis that breaks free, travels through the right side of the heart, and lodges in the lung). It seems that people with VWD should be protected from blood clots, especially blood clots in the veins (deep vein thrombosis or pulmonary embolism), and in most cases people with VWD probably are protected, but there are still circumstances that could precipitate the development of a clot, such as surgery, immobilization, cancer, or too much clotting factor concentrate. Damage to arteries, usually from atherosclerosis, is an important factor in the development of blood clots within the arteries supplying the heart that cause heart attacks or arteries supplying the brain that cause strokes. Risk factors for heart attacks and strokes include high blood pressure, high cholesterol, obesity, smoking, and a family history of heart attacks and strokes. People with VWD can still have risk factors for heart attacks, strokes, and even deep vein thrombosis and pulmonary embolism, but even without these risk factors, it is still possible for a person with VWD to develop a deep vein thrombosis, pulmonary embolism, heart attack, or stroke.

If a person with VWD does develop a deep vein thrombosis, pulmonary embolism, heart attack, or stroke, a hematologist who has expertise in the care of individuals with bleeding disorders should be consulted.

People with VWD can still have risk factors for heart attacks, strokes, and even deep vein thrombosis and pulmonary embolism.

Nikki's story (Type 2B VWD):

With my third child, I hemorrhaged two hours later and had to return to the delivery room, where I was transfused with two units of red blood cells. Ten days later I developed severe pain and swelling in my right leg. The nurse at my doctor's office reassured me that this was normal, even though I couldn't walk on that leg without having severe pain. Finally, after three weeks, the pain and swelling resolved.

The night after the delivery of my fifth child, I knew something was wrong with that leg again. I mentioned it to the obstetrician who took my problem very seriously. He diagnosed me with deep vein thrombosis and started me on heparin (an intravenous anticoagulant). Eight days later, while I was still in the hospital, I developed a pulmonary embolism.

I was in the hospital for another three weeks. After I was discharged, I took Coumadin® (the brand name for the oral anticoagulant warfarin) for six months. During this time, I was in and out of the hospital receiving transfusions of red blood cells and platelets for horrible joint bleeds. This all happened before I knew that I had type 2B VWD.

50. What does my doctor or dentist need to know?

Your doctor or dentist needs to know that you have VWD and what treatment is usually required. He or she may need to contact your hematologist or hemophilia treatment center. Your dentist may need additional information and guidance before he or she performs a dental examination, cleaning, or procedure such as a tooth extraction.

51. Who treats VWD?

Many health care providers are involved in the treatment of patients with VWD, but the doctors who specialize in the treatment of bleeding disorders are hematologists. Hematologists are doctors who completed medical school and then spent another three years training as either a pediatrician or internist (someone who treats adult medical problems). After training as a pediatrician or internist, a hematologist does a three-year fellowship in hematology and oncology. Hematology is the field of medicine that involves the study and treatment of blood disorders, and oncology is the field of medicine that involves the study and treatment of cancer. Sometimes the term "benign hematology" is used to distinguish the study and treatment of blood disorders that are not malignancies or cancers from the study and treatment of blood disorders that are malignancies, such as malignancies of the blood (leukemias) and of the blood-forming organs (lymphomas).

Almost all hematologists in private practice spend more of their time treating cancers than they do treating conditions that are not malignancies such as anemia, sickle cell disease, and bleeding disorders. Hematologists who specialize in treating benign conditions are most often found in university medical centers. Only a few are devoted exclusively to the treatment of bleeding disorders. Doctors who specialize in the treatment of bleeding disorders are most likely to be affiliated with a hemophilia treatment center or other hemostasis center.

52. What is a hemophilia treatment center?

A hemophilia treatment center (HTC) is a clinic where a team of doctors, nurses, social workers, physical therapists, and other specialists work together to deliver comprehensive, state-of-the-art care to people with bleeding disorders. The purpose of comprehensive care is to treat the whole person and his or her family, through supervision of both the medical and psychosocial aspects of bleeding disorders. In comprehensive care, every facet of the person is addressed, including his or her physical, emotional, psychological, educational, financial, and vocational needs. The provision of comprehensive care over the past 30 years has greatly improved the quality of life for people with bleeding disorders and helped them to be more independent and productive. HTCs have lowered patients' morbidity and provided cost-effective care.

The purpose of comprehensive care is to treat the whole person and his or her family, through supervision of both the medical and psychosocial aspects of bleeding disorders.

Having a chronic disease means spending time and energy negotiating the health care system. The staffs at HTCs both help with medical care issues and lend emotional support. Because the staffs at HTCs understand their patients' particular needs, patients use the resources of their HTCs for many years.

Hemophilia treatment centers not only provide specialized care to individuals but can also act as a resource for patients' family physicians or dentists. The staff works closely with local health care providers to meet the specific needs of affected individuals and to improve their quality of life.

Optimal care requires a team of health professionals from several different disciplines.

Von Willebrand disease is a complex condition. Optimal care requires a team of health professionals from several different disciplines. Members of the care team at HTCs include:

- *Adult and pediatric hematologists*—specialists in blood disorders for adults and children.
- *Nurses*—professionals experienced in the care of individuals with bleeding disorders.
- *Social workers*—professionals who assist with the issues of daily living, such as adjusting to the bleeding disorder and locating resources such as insurance, transportation, housing, and so on.
- *Physical therapists*—specialists in activity, exercise, and rehabilitation.
- *Orthopedists*—specialists in disorders of the bones and joints.
- *Dentists*—specialists in disorders of the teeth and gums.

- *Obstetrician gynecologists*—specialists in disorders of the female organs.
- *Coagulation laboratory personnel*—technicians who work behind the scenes performing specialized laboratory tests.

53. Where can I find a hemophilia treatment center?

Care for people with bleeding disorders is provided in different ways in different parts of the world. Some parts of the world do not have the resources even to diagnose bleeding disorders, other parts are able to diagnose bleeding disorders but do not have the full range of treatments, and some parts of the world provide comprehensive care through HTCs.

In the United States

The Maternal Child Health Bureau, of the Health Resources and Services Administration of the Department of Health and Human Services, and the National Centers for Disease Control and Prevention (CDC) support a network of specialized health care centers to prevent and reduce complications experienced by persons with certain blood disorders. Currently, the network includes approximately 140 HTCs. The complete list can be found on the CDC Web site (see Appendix).

In Canada

There are 24 hemophilia treatment centers in Canada. Their locations are listed on the Web site of the Canadian Hemophilia Society (see Appendix).

Worldwide

The World Federation of Hemophilia (WFH) provides a directory of hemophilia treatment centers (HTCs) and hemophilia organizations worldwide on its Web site (see Appendix). This searchable directory, called Passport, is updated daily (as changes are received) and can be used to get a list of all the centers in a country or to find an address of a specific organization or person.

54. Will my insurance company pay for my treatment?

Yes, insurance companies pay for the treatment of VWD. Coverage varies, however. Staffs at HTCs are prepared to counsel you and your family about payment issues.

PART THREE

Women's Issues

How is menorrhagia or heavy menstrual
bleeding managed?

What are hemorrhagic cysts?

Is treatment of VWD safe for an unborn baby?

What is a normal amount of bleeding
after childbirth?

More . . .

55. What is a normal period?

Menstrual periods normally start after age 11 and before age 14. The length of the menstrual cycle is the number of days between the first day of one cycle and the first day of the next cycle. The length of the menstrual cycle should be no shorter than 21 days and no longer than 45 days. A cycle lasting 90 days or longer, in the absence of hormonal treatment, is not normal. A period should last no longer than 7 days. Menstrual flow that requires more than one pad or tampon every hour or two or that results in soaking through night clothes is not normal, nor is passage of clots more than one inch in diameter.

56. What does a girl and her family need to know before her first period?

Girls and their families should know that even the very first menstrual period can be very heavy. Therefore, it would be helpful to discuss the possibility with the girl's doctor in advance and have a plan in place.

Jeanette's story (type 1 VWD with a platelet defect):

I was getting ready to leave the house for a date when I got my first period. Suddenly, my light blue chinos were bright red. Since then, my periods have always been heavy. Stimate® didn't work. I tried going to the hospital for IV DDAVP and that still didn't work. Now I use Humate-P® with uncertain success. So, I worry about my oldest daughter getting her first period. I realize we not only had to have the "talk" about her getting her period and "becoming a woman," but we also had to have the talk about her getting her period and having a bleeding disorder. CSL Behring and our local hemophilia treatment center sponsored a mother-daughter luncheon at a restaurant in our community. The luncheon was a beautiful way to introduce the subject.

57. What is menorrhagia?

Menorrhagia is the medical term for heavy menstrual bleeding. It refers specifically to *regular* heavy menstrual bleeding, as opposed to *irregular* heavy menstrual bleeding. The term menometrorrhagia includes irregular heavy menstrual bleeding, but the term is rarely used. More often, the term menorrhagia is used for all heavy menstrual bleeding, both regular and irregular. Menorrhagia is defined as the passage of more than 80 milliliters of blood per month. This is approximately one-third of a cup. Outside of research studies, no one actually measures menstrual blood flow, but the loss of 80 milliliters of blood per month correlates with soaking through more than one pad or tampon per hour, soaking through bed clothes at night, and passing clots one inch in diameter or more. The loss of 80 milliliters of blood per month can also result in low iron levels or anemia.

Menorrhagia
Heavy menstrual bleeding.

Women with VWD are more likely to have heavy menstrual bleeding or menorrhagia. In various medical reports, 32% to 100% of women with VWD experienced heavy menstrual bleeding. In other medical reports of women with heavy menstrual bleeding, 5% to 20% were found to have previously undiagnosed VWD.

Women with VWD are more likely to have heavy menstrual bleeding or menorrhagia.

58. What else causes heavy menstrual bleeding?

There are other causes of heavy menstrual bleeding besides VWD and other bleeding disorders. One other cause is anovulation or lack of ovulation. Ovulation is the process that results in the release of an egg or ovum from an ovary. The two ovaries are the reproductive organs in a female that produce eggs or ova. Eggs or ova, when fertilized by sperm from a male, become embryos that can develop into a fetus and ultimately a baby. In most menstrual cycles, ovulation occurs approximately two weeks from the start of a woman's or girl's last menstrual period. During the early part of the menstrual cycle, the lining of the uterus, or endometrium, builds up in preparation for a possible pregnancy. At the time of ovulation, the ovum is released, and its sac produces the hormone progesterone. Progesterone matures the lining of the uterus in preparation for a possible pregnancy. If pregnancy does not occur, the mature endometrium is shed in an organized way. If ovulation does not occur, the lining of the uterus or endometrium can continue to build up until the blood supply from the uterus cannot sustain the endometrium any longer and it is shed intermittently in a disorganized way. This can result in very heavy menstrual bleeding. Anovulation or lack of ovulation is more likely to affect girls just starting to menstruate and women approaching menopause. Other causes of anovulation include low levels of thyroid hormone and a condition known as polycystic ovarian disease.

Conditions that affect the lining of the uterus or endometrium can also cause heavy menstrual bleeding.

Conditions that affect the lining of the uterus or endometrium can also cause heavy menstrual bleeding. These conditions include fibroids (benign tumors of the uterus), polyps (abnormal growths arising from the glands of the uterus), endometrial hyperplasia (overgrowth of the lining of the uterus), and even cancer. These conditions rarely affect girls and young women but can affect women who are in their thirties or older. Therefore, a medical evaluation of menorrhagia or heavy menstrual bleeding in women in their thirties or older will often include not only a pelvic examination and Pap smear but an ultrasound to look for fibroids, polyps, or endometrial hyperplasia, and a biopsy to make sure that no cancer is present.

59. How is menorrhagia or heavy menstrual bleeding managed?

If a girl or woman has menorrhagia, the full range of treatments to manage heavy menstrual bleeding may be tried. The girl or woman should first be evaluated by a gynecologist to make sure there is no abnormality of the uterus or its lining (endometrium). An ultrasound of the uterus may be performed. If an abnormality of the uterus or its lining (endometrium) is detected, minor surgery may be required to correct the abnormality. A biopsy of the endometrium may be performed to make sure there is no cancer or precancerous condition, especially if a woman is in her thirties or older. If there is no abnormality, hormonal treatments may be tried. Birth control pills, patches and rings, and the Mirena® intra-uterine device (IUD) reduce heavy periods, and thus may be prescribed. Birth control pills, patches, and rings are useful not only because they reduce menstrual blood flow but also because they contain estrogen, which can raise von Willebrand factor and factor VIII levels. Some women who stop taking birth control pills notice that they have more bruises and experience more bleeding.

There are other options for the woman who does not plan to have any more children. She may have the lining of her uterus destroyed by a technique called endometrial ablation or even undergo a hysterectomy. Endometrial ablation can reduce or eliminate menstruation. However, one out of every five to ten procedures is unsuccessful, and one out of three women ultimately undergoes a hysterectomy. Hysterectomy, an operation to remove the uterus, is major surgery and requires special planning (see Question 46).

60. Is it safe to have a hysterectomy?

If proper precautions are taken, it is safe to have a hysterectomy, but a woman with menorrhagia should not undergo a hysterectomy until all other appropriate options have been tried. A hysterectomy is major surgery. Therefore, women with VWD should insist on having their operation at a medical center with a hemophilia treatment center or similar hemostasis center. This center should have a laboratory capable of performing specialized coagulation tests 24 hours a day, a pharmacy with von Willebrand factor concentrates, and a knowledgeable hematologist, surgeon, and anesthesiologist. Prior to major surgery, von Willebrand ristocetin cofactor activity (VWF:RCo) and factor VIII levels should be at least 100 IU/dL. These levels should be maintained for at least 7 to 14 days. These levels will usually require factor replacement with VWF concentrates. Close monitoring is required to prevent levels from dropping below 50 IU/dL, which would increase the risk of bleeding, or from rising above 200 to 300 IU/dL, which would increase the risk of abnormal blood clots.

61. What is "dysmenorrhea"?

Dysmenorrhea

Painful menstruation.

Although some pain during menstruation is normal, excessive pain is not.

Dysmenorrhea is the medical term for painful menstrual periods. Although some pain during menstruation is normal, excessive pain is not. Menstrual periods may be accompanied by crampy lower abdominal pain. A woman may feel sharp pain that comes and goes or have dull, aching pain. Menstrual periods may also cause back pain. The pain may begin several days before, or just at the start of, a period and generally subsides as menstrual bleeding tapers off.

Painful menstrual periods or dysmenorrhea affects many women. For some women and girls, such discomfort makes it nearly impossible to perform normal activities for a few days during each menstrual cycle. Painful menstruation is the leading cause of time lost from school and work among women and girls in their teens and twenties.

Activity of the hormone prostaglandin, produced in the uterus, is thought to be a factor in dysmenorrhea. The hormone prostaglandin causes contraction of the uterus. Prostaglandin levels tend to be much higher in women and girls with severe menstrual pain than in women who experience mild or no menstrual pain. The most common and most effective treatment for dysmenorrhea is non-steroidal anti-inflammatory drugs (NSAIDs) such as ibuprofen (Motrin®), naproxen (Aleve®, and mefenamic acid (Ponstel®). These drugs inhibit prostaglandins. They may also affect the function of platelets and interfere with normal blood clotting (see Question 2). Since aspirin and other NSAIDs can increase the tendency to bleed, individuals with VWD are generally counseled to avoid these medications.

Unfortunately, women and girls with VWD seem to be more likely to experience painful menstrual periods. This may be because their periods tend to be heavier. Choices of pain medication are limited to acetaminophen (Tylenol®), narcotics such as codeine, oxycodone, and hydrocodone, and an occasional dose of an NSAID.

62. What is Mittelschmerz?

Mittelschmerz is a German word for "middle pain" and is used to describe the pain that sometimes accompanies ovulation. Ovulation is the process that results in the release of an egg or ovum from an ovary, the reproductive organ that produces eggs or ova, in a woman or girl. (Eggs or ova, if fertilized by sperm from a male, become embryos that can develop into a fetus and ultimately a baby.) In most menstrual cycles, approximately two weeks from the start of the last menstrual period, a woman or girl ovulates. When ovulation occurs, the ovum actually breaks through the surface of the ovary. Ovulation is not normally accompanied by any pain or bleeding, but in a woman or girl with VWD, the potential exists for bleeding and pain.

63. What are hemorrhagic cysts?

Hemorrhagic ovarian cysts result from bleeding at the time of ovulation. Ovulation is not normally accompanied by any significant amount of bleeding, but in a woman with VWD, the potential exists for bleeding into the ovary, forming a hemorrhagic cyst, or bleeding into the abdomen. Combined hormonal contraceptives that contain a combination of estrogen and progestin (a synthetic progesterone) effectively prevent ovulation and prevent bleeding into the ovary or abdomen. This is another reason why women with VWD should be encouraged to use combined hormonal contraceptives such as birth control pills, patches, or rings.

Vicki's story (type 3 VWD):

At 13, I became a "WOMAN." I started my periods quite normally, exactly 12 months after my sister, who was 13 months older than me. My periods lasted 3 to 5 days and I could predict the date and time that they would start, at 10 a.m. on the twenty-eighth day. Pretty predictable, huh? The part I could not predict was the incredible pain and discomfort that occurred halfway between my periods. The only explanation that the OB/GYN could give was that I was bruising when the egg popped from the ovary. At 16, and suffering with this every other month for three years, I was put on the pill at a time when good girls did not have to be on contraceptives. The pills helped control the issue and I stayed on them for the next seven years until my husband and I decided to try for a child.

64. What can be used for birth control?

All methods of birth control can be used, but some methods, such as the copper IUD (ParaGard®), tend to increase menstrual bleeding and should be avoided. Others result in decreased bleeding and are preferred. Combined hormonal contraceptives, which contain a combination of estrogen and progestin (a synthetic progesterone), prevent ovulation, prevent hemorrhagic ovarian cysts, and tend to reduce heavy menstrual bleeding. Therefore, combined hormonal contraceptives, such as birth control pills, patches, or rings, are a good choice. Progestin-only contraceptives such as progestin-only birth control pills (Micronor®, Nor-QD®, and Ovrette®), the Depo-Provera® injections, the Implanon® implant, and the Mirena® IUD also reduce heavy menstrual bleeding. There is a new formulation of the Depo-Provera® injection that allows it to be injected into the fatty tissue under the skin rather than into the muscle, making it safer for women with VWD. The Implanon® implant has to be inserted under the skin, which can cause bleeding, so it may not be a good choice. The Mirena® IUD has been shown to be effective at reducing menstrual bleeding in women with VWD and therefore is a good alternative.

65. Is it normal for a woman with VWD to have bleeding with sexual intercourse?

No, it is not normal for a woman with VWD to have bleeding with sexual intercourse.

Normal, healthy tissue in the vagina and on the cervix (the opening to the uterus) does not bleed. Bleeding with sexual intercourse may be a sign of an abnormality and should always be investigated by a gynecologist. There are times in a woman's life, however, that she may experience small tears in her vagina with intercourse. These tears could bleed. A woman is actually vulnerable to small tears when her vagina has been deprived of estrogen and the tissue is thin. This condition occurs after childbirth and again after menopause. It is treatable with estrogen. Another time in a woman's life when she is vulnerable to bleeding with sexual relations is at the time of first intercourse, when the hymen, or membrane around the opening of the vagina, is torn. This can result in significant bleeding and young women with VWD should be warned.

Vicki's story (type 3 VWD):

I married at 18, the day after I graduated from high school, much to the dismay of my parents and David's. My parents had planned for me to go to college and graduate school to become a doctor. David's mother could just not understand why he would want to marry a girl so ill. David was in the Navy and we immediately moved to Norfolk, VA. My wedding night, I started my period, or so I thought. After 10 days of bleeding and by then feeling quite ill, we went to the military hospital and sat in the clinic for three hours. I was feeling very weak and dizzy by then. My young, newly enlisted husband went into the hall and commandeered one of the doctors (who were officers) and nearly dragged him into the clinic. Well, they took me next and as soon as I passed through the doors from the waiting area, I fainted. Talk about getting help: when I came to, there were three doctors, four nurses, and one very frightened new husband surrounding me on the floor. I learned then that when you lose your virginity, you also tear your hymen, and a person with VWD might bleed.

Andra's story (low VWF or mild type 1 VWD):

I went to bed the night after my first sexual relations and woke up early the next morning in a puddle of blood. Unlike Vicki, I had no further bleeding. I have since learned that most women do not experience that amount of bleeding with first sexual relations, but many women with VWD have been similarly surprised.

66. What is endometriosis?

Endometriosis is the presence of patches of endometrial tissue, the tissue that lines the uterus, in the abdomen outside of the uterus. Endometriosis can cause severe abdominal pain, especially when the patches of endometrial tissue swell under the influence of the hormones of the menstrual cycle. In a survey of 102 women with VWD, 30% reported a history of endometriosis compared with 13% of women without VWD. There are several possible reasons why women with VWD would be more likely to be diagnosed with endometriosis. Although there is disagreement about what causes endometriosis, the main theory is that it results from retrograde menstruation, menstruation that flows backward from the uterus out of the fallopian tubes into the abdomen. Retrograde menstruation is more likely to occur during heavy menstrual periods. Women with VWD are certainly more likely to experience heavy menstrual periods. Another possible

Endometriosis

The presence of patches of endometrial tissue, the tissue that lines the uterus, in the abdomen.

There are several possible reasons why women with VWD would be more likely to be diagnosed with endometriosis.

reason why women with VWD would be more likely to be diagnosed with endometriosis is that women with VWD may be more likely to experience bleeding from the patches of endometrial tissue that have escaped the uterus. A third possible reason is that women with VWD are more likely to experience hemorrhagic ovarian cysts or bleeding into the abdomen that may be incorrectly diagnosed as endometriosis.

Endometriosis is diagnosed during a surgical procedure that allows the gynecologist to see the inside of the abdomen. The procedure is usually performed with a laparoscope, a lighted instrument that is inserted into the abdomen through a small incision. Endometriosis is treated by eradicating the patches during surgery or by suppressing the patches with hormones.

Vicki's story (type 3 VWD):

At 23, in 1981, we decided to get pregnant, so I came off birth control. Within months, I was having the mid-cycle pain again. I dealt with it. I was used to it. I had no clue that it would affect pregnancy. After a few months, the pain was getting worse and I started to feel weak and dizzy. Off to the doctor again. We were stationed in Boston during this time and living in Quincy, MA. There was no military hospital, so I went to the community health center I had aligned with and had an exam. I remember that it was winter and getting dark; the doctor looked at me and said I needed to go immediately to the hospital, no ifs, buts, or wherefores. David was at work, the hospital was downtown Boston and the doctor did not even want me to go home and let the dog out or pack a bag. Well, I talked him into letting me go home, pack a bag, and get my husband to drive me downtown. I think the doctor even had a problem finding a hospital that had a bed that could take me.

I ended up at Tufts/New England Medical Center. Again, I was anemic, but this time I had a mass the size of a grapefruit in my abdomen. The doctors feared a tumor. I was worked up for exploratory surgery, a new technique called laparoscopy with the potential for a full hysterectomy. I was scared to death and only 23, but fine, these were the best doctors and I trusted them. After the work up, the team of doctors came in and said that the surgery had been cancelled because they could not get my bleeding time into normal range and could therefore not take me safely into the operating room. I was crushed. I had resigned myself to the fact that I was having a hysterectomy, that pregnancy would never happen, and that adoption proceedings would take place immediately upon my release from the hospital. Adoption had always been discussed, particularly between my husband and my mother.

The next problem was dealing with the mass in my abdomen. They really thought I had cancer. I really thought it had something to do with VWD. They couldn't go in there and look and I could not keep going with it in me. The doctors decided to try a new medication, Danazol, which was still in medical trials for endometriosis. They said that if it was a blood mass or endometriosis, this medication should decrease the mass immediately, by stopping all menstrual activity. If it were a tumor, the Danazol would not do anything and they would have to put their heads together to figure out something else. The medication was approved for six months of use; I was on it for ten months. After the first month or two, the doctors saw a definite decrease in the mass, ergo, it must be endometriosis. During this time the discussion of pregnancy was again raised, by me of course. I spoke with my doctors and was told that once I stopped the Danazol, I would be in the best position to get pregnant and that pregnancy would help keep any further endometriosis away. I was also told that delivery would not be an issue, because "the hospital had plenty of blood in the blood bank"!!

After being on the Danazol, I expected to get pregnant within the next six months. After three months I started having mid-cycle pain again and knew that the endometriosis had come back. Back onto the Danazol for another few months, and David and I determined that natural childbirth was not in the cards for us. I started continuous hormone therapy and have been on one type or another ever since. During that summer of recuperation, I was not allowed to pick up or do anything. I read, learned to crochet, and got a new job at a bank in the fall. I took what I learned with us to our next duty station. I started work at another bank, we bought our first home, and in 1985 we filed papers for an adoption home study. We began an adoption support group for couples on the adoption waiting list and bided our time. In 1989, we were blessed with a baby girl only two-and-a-half weeks old.

67. What if a woman wants to become pregnant?

Ideally, planning for pregnancy begins before conception. Women contemplating a pregnancy should be aware that they may be at an increased risk of bleeding complications. Prior to conception or during pregnancy, women may want to take the opportunity to speak with a genetic counselor regarding the inheritance of VWD, and with a pediatric hematologist regarding the evaluation of the infant after delivery. Because of the possible need for transfusion, women who have not already been vaccinated should be immunized against hepatitis A and hepatitis B. Few options are available to prevent menorrhagia and Mittelschmerz or hemorrhagic ovarian cysts in women who are trying to conceive. Hormones interfere with or prevent conception and should not be used, but DDAVP, antifibrinolytics, or a VWF/FVIII concentrate may be tried.

During pregnancy, levels of von Willebrand factor increase. Women with mild type 1 may achieve levels above 50 IU/dL, the lower limit of the normal range outside of pregnancy, and may be able to be safely delivered at their local hospital.

Women with type 3 VWD, type 2 VWD, or type 1 VWD with factor VIII levels less than 50 IU/dL, a von Willebrand ristocetin cofactor activity (VWF:RCo) less than 50 IU/dL, or a history of severe bleeding should be referred for prenatal care and delivery to a center where, in addition to specialists in high-risk obstetrics, there is a hemophilia treatment center or a hematologist with expertise in VWD. Laboratory, pharmacy, and blood bank support is essential. Prior to any procedure that could result in bleeding such as chorionic villus sampling, amniocentesis, or cervical cerclage, these women should receive prophylaxis against bleeding. Factor VIII and VWF:RCo levels should be obtained and repeated in the third trimester of pregnancy to facilitate planning for delivery.

Factor VIII and VWF:RCo levels should be obtained and repeated in the third trimester of pregnancy to facilitate planning for delivery.

68. What are the risks of a pregnancy?

Besides all of the usual risks of pregnancy, the risks to a woman with VWD include bleeding during the pregnancy and **postpartum hemorrhage**. Despite the fact that von Willebrand factor and factor VIII levels rise during pregnancy, they may not rise to the same extent that they do in a woman without VWD.

Postpartum hemorrhage

Excessive bleeding after childbirth.

69. Is treatment of VWD safe for an unborn baby?

DDAVP, if required prior to a procedure, is generally thought to be safe for the mother and her unborn baby.

Tranexamic acid crosses the placenta but has been used to treat bleeding during pregnancy in a limited number of cases without adverse fetal effects. There are limited data about aminocaproic acid (Amicar) in pregnancy, but it was not found to cause birth defects in rabbits and in one case of its use during pregnancy, there were also no adverse fetal effects.

Von Willebrand Factor concentrates, derived from purified human plasma, carry a theoretical risk of virus transmission. During the purification process, viruses are inactivated, including potentially harmful viruses. While the risk of virus transmission exists, because of improved selection of plasma donors, testing of donated plasma, and improved virus inactivation processes, no transmission of human immunodeficiency virus (HIV), hepatitis B, or hepatitis C have occurred with any VWF concentrates currently marketed in the United States. Parvovirus B19, however, is very difficult to eradicate despite the purification process. Parvovirus B19 can cause a mild disease (fever, rash, aches, and pains) in adults, but can cause severe, life-threatening anemia in unborn babies. There is a risk that this virus could be transmitted even with purified factor products and harm a fetus. There are no reports of this actually happening, however.

Blood products such as fresh frozen plasma and cryoprecipitate are tested for known viruses, but are not purified and may allow unknown, potentially harmful viruses to be transmitted.

70. What is a normal amount of bleeding after childbirth?

Bleeding is normal after childbirth. The average amount of blood lost after a vaginal delivery is 500 milliliters, or approximately a pint. The average amount of blood lost at the time of a cesarean delivery is 1,000 milliliters, or approximately a quart.

71. What is a postpartum hemorrhage?

A postpartum hemorrhage is excessive blood loss at the time of childbirth. The definition of postpartum hemorrhage is 500 milliliters, which, ironically, is the average amount of blood lost at the time of a vaginal delivery. Women make and store extra blood during pregnancy, so the loss of 500 to 1,000 milliliters at the time of delivery does not cause any serious problems. Women are more likely to perceive that they have had a hemorrhage than are their doctors or midwives. Twenty percent of women report that they have had a postpartum hemorrhage at the time of delivery, whereas physicians or midwives make the diagnosis only 4 percent of the time. In women with VWD, the diagnosis is made 6 percent of the time. Loss of more than 1,000 milliliters can cause symptoms of anemia, and loss of more than 1,500 milliliters can cause symptoms of severe anemia or shock. One percent of women require a blood transfusion at the time of childbirth, whereas 1.5 percent of women with VWD require transfusion.

Women are more likely to perceive that they have had a hemorrhage than are their doctors or midwives.

72. What causes postpartum hemorrhage?

Most postpartum hemorrhage is caused by failure of the uterus to contract or tighten after delivery. After a child is born, the placenta (afterbirth) separates and is delivered. The placenta is about the size of a plate. The space on the inside of the uterus that was occupied by the placenta is filled with numerous open blood vessels. To prevent hemorrhage, these blood vessels must constrict to prevent blood loss and the uterus must contract to promote blood vessel constriction. Prior to delivery, approximately 750 milliliters, or three quarters of a quart of blood, flow through the uterus every minute. Without contraction of the uterus, massive hemorrhage can occur. Women with or without a bleeding disorder can suffer from this type of hemorrhage.

Women with a bleeding disorder are particularly vulnerable to delayed postpartum hemorrhage.

Women with a bleeding disorder are particularly vulnerable to delayed postpartum hemorrhage, the type that occurs more than 24 hours after childbirth. This type of hemorrhage occurs after less than one percent of deliveries, but occurs in up to 25 percent of women with a bleeding disorder. Normal blood clotting appears to be necessary to prevent delayed postpartum hemorrhage.

Jeanette's story (type 1 VWD with a platelet defect):

After each of my children was born, I had a postpartum hemorrhage. By then, we knew my diagnosis. VWF concentrates were not available to me due to insurance issues, but my local hematologists arranged for my husband to give plasma so that I could receive direct-donor cryo, should I need it. This was done for all three of my pregnancies. With some of these delayed postpartum hemorrhages, in addition to receiving medications to make my uterus contract, such as Pitocin® (oxytocin) and Methergine® (methylergonovine maleate), I was able to receive his direct-donor cryo and didn't have to receive any other transfusions. Because I needed to be near the hospital in case I needed my husband's direct-donor cryo, I wasn't able to leave the area for three to four months after each delivery.

Having a child should be a joyful time, not a fearful time. All women fear childbirth, but women with bleeding disorders are especially fearful of having a hemorrhage. They should understand that bleeding can be managed, that hemorrhage can be prevented, and that they can have a safe, successful delivery.

73. How is postpartum hemorrhage prevented in a woman with VWD?

The most important measure in preventing postpartum hemorrhage is recognizing the possibility that it can happen. Doctors and midwives anticipate the possibility with every delivery. In modern hospitals and birthing centers, an intravenous catheter (a tube in the vein) is inserted prior to delivery. This allows for the administration of medications, fluids, and blood, if necessary. Doctors and midwives actively manage the third stage of labor, the period of time from delivery of the infant to delivery of the placenta. The natural hormone that causes the uterus to contract, oxytocin, is given intravenously. Before and after the placenta is delivered, the uterus is massaged to help it contract.

The most important measure in preventing postpartum hemorrhage is recognizing the possibility that it can happen.

To help prevent bleeding from tears and incisions and to prevent delayed postpartum hemorrhage, women with VWD need to have at least 50 percent of normal levels of von Willebrand factor and factor VIII. Prior to delivery, and for the first few days after delivery, von Willebrand ristocetin cofactor activity (VWF:RCo) and factor VIII levels should be at least 100 IU/dL. Like after major surgery, close monitoring is required to prevent factor levels from dropping below 50 IU/dL, which would increase the risk of bleeding, or from rising above 200 to 300 IU/dL, which would increase the risk of abnormal blood clots. Sufficient levels will usually require factor replacement with VWF concentrates. DDAVP is a synthetic version of the hormone vasopressin, an "antidiuretic" hormone. It can cause water to be retained, diluting the blood and lowering the concentration of sodium, an essential mineral. This is more likely to occur when repeated doses are necessary or fluids cannot be restricted, which is the case at the time of childbirth when several liters of fluid are administered. Also, the hormone oxytocin, which is chemically very similar to the hormone vasopressin, can also cause water to be retained. DDAVP must be used with extreme caution at the time of childbirth, or a dangerously low concentration of sodium could result in seizures.

74. How is postpartum hemorrhage managed in a woman with VWD?

Doctors' and midwives' first response to postpartum hemorrhage is stimulating the uterus to contract. This is accomplished with massage and with the hormone oxytocin. They will also make sure that the uterus is empty, allowing it to contract better. This may require the removal of blood clots or fragments of placenta. Doctors' and midwives' next response is administering additional medications to cause the uterus to contract. In some cases, emergency surgery may be necessary to scrape the uterus (curettage), physically compress the uterus (bimanual compression), or tie off (ligate) blood vessels. Hysterectomy is a last resort and is only necessary after 1 in 1,000 deliveries.

Every effort will be made to ensure that VWF levels are sufficient to prevent bleeding from tears and incisions and to prevent delayed postpartum hemorrhage. In the case of massive hemorrhage, blood products may be necessary.

75. Can women with VWD have an epidural or spinal anesthetic at the time of delivery?

An epidural anesthetic provides pain relief during labor. To administer this medication, a catheter (thin tube) is placed into the epidural space, which is just outside of the dura, or wrapping, around the spinal cord; repeated or continuous doses of a local anesthetic or narcotic pain reliever are then delivered through this catheter. In contrast, a spinal anesthetic provides anesthesia for cesarean delivery. Administration of a spinal anesthetic involves a single injection of a local anesthetic into the spinal fluid, which is located beneath the dura and surrounds the spinal cord. Because bleeding in the epidural space or spinal fluid could compress the spine and cause paralysis, anesthesiologists usually refrain from giving a patient with VWD an epidural or spinal anesthetic unless her factor VIII and von Willebrand ristocetin cofactor activity (VWF:RCo) levels are continuously higher than 50 IU/dL. If a woman needs pain relief in labor and does not have factor VIII and VWF:RCo levels that are continuously higher than 50 IU/dL, narcotic pain relievers can be used instead of an epidural. If she requires a cesarean delivery, a general anesthetic can be used instead of a spinal.

In the case of massive hemorrhage, blood products may be necessary.

76. What about the baby?

The baby of a mother or father with VWD has a 50 percent chance of being affected with the condition. Except in cases where a severely affected infant is expected, the baby can be safely born through the vagina. There is a risk to infants who are severely affected with type 3 VWD of having a hemorrhage in the brain at the time of birth. The risk of hemorrhage in the brain is increased with a vaginal delivery, especially if forceps or vacuum extraction is used. Rarely, however, is the diagnosis suspected before delivery. Except for type 3 and type 2N, which are transmitted by recessive inheritance, an infant has a 50% chance of being affected and affected with the same type of VWD as his or her affected parent. Therefore, general precautions are taken at the time of childbirth whenever there is a potentially affected infant. These precautions include avoiding invasive procedures such as placement of an internal fetal scalp monitor or delivery by forceps or vacuum extraction. Circumcision is a strictly elective (not medically necessary) procedure that should be postponed until the infant boy's von Willebrand factor level has been determined and is sufficient. If the infant does not have sufficient VWF and is found to have VWD, he will require VWF replacement before undergoing circumcision or can forego this strictly elective procedure.

Because VWF levels at birth can be influenced by many factors and may not accurately reflect whether an infant has VWD or not, tests for VWD are usually repeated at 6 months of age.

Jeanette's story (type 1 VWD with a platelet defect):

Because we knew my son might have VWD, we chose not to have him circumcised when he was a newborn. Six months later, when he was tested, he turned out to have VWD, so we decided not to have him circumcised. When he was 5 years old, his foreskin was stuck and we wound up having to have him circumcised. He was pretreated with DDAVP and did fine.

PART FOUR

Managing Other Bleeding Symptoms

What if there is blood in my urine?

What if I get a nosebleed?

Can von Willebrand disease cause joint bleeds?

More . . .

77. What if there is blood in my urine?

Blood in the urine is not normal. The medical term for red blood cells in the urine is hematuria. Sometimes what someone thinks is blood in the urine is merely a discoloration due to beets or is blood from the vagina or rectum. Blood in the urine can be a sign of a serious problem in the urinary tract (bladder, ureters, or kidneys). Hematuria can result from infection, inflammation, or injury to the urinary tract. Only after a thorough evaluation by a health care provider should blood in the urine be attributed to VWD. If the blood is significant and your health care provider is not readily available, you should go to a hospital emergency room.

Blood in the urine can be a sign of a serious problem in the urinary tract.

78. What if there is bleeding at the time of a bowel movement?

Bleeding at the time of a bowel movement is not normal. Bleeding is a sign that there is a tear or a more serious problem somewhere along the intestinal tract. Usually, the problem is only a tear around the rectal opening and will heal on its own, but bleeding that is excessive or persists for days requires medical attention. Bleeding that might be trivial in a person without a bleeding disorder can be life threatening in a person with VWD.

Tears are more likely to occur if there is constipation or straining to move bowels. Everyone, but especially those with bleeding disorders, should avoid constipation and avoid straining to move bowels. You can avoid constipation by drinking water and fluids and by taking a daily stool softener (a medication which softens bowel movements), such as Colace®. If constipation does occur, you may try a mild laxative (a medication that stimulates bowel movements) after checking with your doctor or nurse.

Vicki's story (type 3 VWD):

In 1992, when I got sick again, and the doctor determined that I was having some bleeding in my gastrointestinal tract, I was moved from the military hospital to a hospital downtown and given a horrible set of gastrointestinal (GI) tract tests. Back then, you had to drink what seemed like five gallons of horrible-tasting liquid, and when you are already ill, this does not go down well. I was also given two bags of cryoprecipitate and was told it was equivalent to 75 units of plasma. This was to prepare me for laparoscopic exploratory surgery. That too was cancelled due to the fact that they could not bring my bleeding into acceptable limits.

I have had a total of three gastrointestinal bleeds. The first I did not recognize and was hospitalized for a few days, given two units of blood, had to do the horrid GI tests again and was infused for a week after. The second I recognized quicker, infused at home, and had a small drop in hemoglobin and hematocrit after outpatient testing. The third I recognized within hours with no problems after only one infusion.

79. How can I prevent gum bleeding?

Gum disease is caused by plaque, a sticky film of bacteria that constantly forms on the teeth. These bacteria create toxins that damage the gums and cause bleeding. When plaque has hardened on the teeth, it is necessary for a dental hygienist or a dentist to scrape this material off. Gum bleeding is much less likely to occur with healthy gums. To maintain healthy gums:

- Brush your teeth after every meal.
- Visit the dentist or dental hygienist twice a year for dental cleaning.
- Floss your teeth at least once a day.

- Decrease the quantity and frequency of your sugar. Sugar helps plaque grow.
- Consider using a use a high-quality electric toothbrush.

To prevent additional bleeding when bleeding is a problem:

- Use a soft toothbrush. A soft toothbrush treats the gums more gently so they are less likely to bleed.
- Hold off on the flossing until the bleeding subsides.
- Eat a soft diet, such as soup, mashed potatoes, custards, gelatin, or pudding. Avoid foods that are sharp or crunchy or are very hot. Soft foods are less likely to cause cuts or sores. Very hot foods can cause burns that can blister and bleed.

Vicki's story (type 3 VWD):

I remember the first cleaning I had with one dentist in Jacksonville, Florida. The hygienist cleaned so well that my mouth was filled with blood. I told her not to worry, that it happened all the time, it would stop . . . eventually. The doctor came in and I thought he might pass out, he stammered that he had never seen anything like that and he could not do an exam as he could not see anything through the blood. He asked me to come back in a week. I did, we talked about my bleeding again (I had talked about it before the cleaning) and we decided that I would not floss, make sure that I brushed very well, and increased my cleanings to three times a year. I loved that dentist, shocked though he was at first. We left Jacksonville in 1981, but went back in 1985. I returned to that dentist and stayed with him until we moved in 1993. I still brush very well with a motorized toothbrush and get three cleanings per year. I infuse before each and every dental visit and no longer bleed afterwards.

80. What if mouth bleeding is severe?

- If mouth bleeding is severe, apply steady pressure for a full 15 minutes. Use a clock to time the 15 minutes. It can seem like a long time. Resist the urge to peek after a few minutes to see whether bleeding has stopped. If blood soaks through the cloth, apply another one without lifting the first.

- For inner lip bleeding, press the bleeding site against the teeth or jaw or place a rolled or folded piece of gauze or clean cloth between the lip and gum. Once bleeding from inside the lip stops, don't pull the lip out again to look at it. Avoid yawning or laughing, which may make the bleeding begin again.

- For tongue bleeding, squeeze or press the bleeding site with gauze or a piece of clean cloth.

- For inner cheek bleeding, place rolled gauze or a piece of clean cloth between the wound and the teeth.

- For bleeding after tooth extraction, follow any instructions from the dentist. Bite on gauze or a piece of clean cloth to control bleeding. If pressure does not stop the bleeding, try biting down on a moistened tea bag for 10 to 15 minutes. Avoid spitting, using any form of tobacco, and using straws, which can make the bleeding worse.

81. What if I get a nosebleed?

Sit up. Do not lie down. Lying down increases the amount of blood flowing to the head and can aggravate the bleeding. Bend forward slightly. This prevents blood from dripping down the back of the throat and causing gagging. Apply direct pressure by pinching the nostrils together for 10 to 15 minutes. At the same time breathe through the mouth and spit all blood and saliva into sink or a bowl. Place an ice pack over the bridge of the nose.

This will cause blood vessels to tighten or constrict and prevent additional bleeding. Most nosebleeds will stop with direct pressure. Seek medical attention if the nosebleed does not stop in 10 to 15 minutes. Nosebleeds that do not stop in 10 to 15 minutes may require treatment to raise von Willebrand factor levels, antifibrinolytic medication, cauterization of the bleeding blood vessel or vessels (which are usually located on the nasal septum or membrane between the nostrils), or packing of the nose with gauze. While the bleeding is occurring, do not administer nasal DDAVP (Stimate®) in the affected nostril or nostrils. Rest to help prevent further bleeding.

Most people, even with VWD, outgrow their nosebleeds or have fewer nosebleeds when they become adults.

Most people, even with VWD, outgrow their nosebleeds or have fewer nosebleeds when they become adults.

Garry's story (type 2A VWD):

I have had nosebleeds my entire life. For thirty years, I did body work and the dust was very irritating. Just about every day that I worked, I had nosebleeds. I had my nose cauterized in the 1980s, but that didn't cure the problem. One thing I have learned is how to pack a nose. I use a combination of gauze and styptic powder. (Styptic powder is an antiseptic clotting agent that is most often used in pet grooming. Much like a styptic pencil, which is made of alum, styptic powder stops bleeding by contracting blood vessels.)

Vicki's story (type 3 VWD):

I have to give my local doctors credit for being very innovative in treating my VWD. The ear, nose, and throat doctor found this special cotton packing called Oxycel® by Parke-Davis to pack my nose with when it bled. This cotton was treated with oxidized cellulose and once inserted would swell from the blood, stop the bleeding, and after two to three days dissolve, fall out, and not start the bleeding again. I used Oxycel® until my late teens/early twenties. My mom packed my nose and then by the time I was twelve I was packing my nose myself.

By the time I was an adult, my nosebleeds had pretty much gone away. I still have them in the cold and dry weather, but a humidifier by the bed helps.

82. How can nosebleeds be prevented?

Limit activity for a day or two. Vigorous exercise can cause nosebleeds to recur, so it is best to refrain from vigorous activity for a day or two after a nosebleed. Avoid heavy lifting and avoid straining to have a bowel movement.

Keep the inside of the nose lubricated. A little dab of petroleum jelly placed over the irritated area on the inside of the nose for a few days may help prevent bleeding.

Keep the moist membranes of the nose from drying out. Invest in a humidifier. Since one of the most common causes of nosebleeds is dryness of the moist membranes that line the nose, breathing well-humidified air may help protect against some nosebleeds. Saline nose spray can also help keep the membranes moist.

Avoid trauma to the nose. Blow gently. Keep objects, including fingers, out of the nose.

Minimize nasal discharge. Antihistamines can reduce nasal discharge from allergies.

Make sure your blood pressure is normal. High blood pressure can increase the chance of having a nosebleed.

Do not smoke. Besides many other harmful consequences of smoking, smoking increases the chance of having a nosebleed.

Make sure that you are not taking a medication that increases the risk of bleeding (see Question 86).

83. *Are bruises a cause for concern?*

When the soft tissues under the skin are injured, the small veins or venules and capillaries, the thinnest, tiniest blood vessels, can leak. After hemoglobin, the molecule in the red blood cells that carries oxygen in the blood and gives blood its red color, leaks into the soft tissues, the hemoglobin changes color from red to purple to blue or even black. When the hemoglobin accumulates under the skin, it leaves a "black-and-blue mark." Bruises go through colorful changes as the hemoglobin is processed into a form the body can get rid of. The hemoglobin is converted into substances called bile pigments that are initially green and ultimately yellow in color.

Bruises are not harmful in and of themselves.

Bruises are not harmful in and of themselves. They arise from blood that is contained under the skin and do not pose a risk to internal organs. They are merely a sign of a bleeding tendency. They pose a problem only if bleeding is severe. Severe bleeding into a muscle can cause a condition known as compartment syndrome in which the accumulated blood puts pressure on blood vessels, interferes with circulation, and deprives muscles of oxygen. This condition results in a painful, swollen arm or leg and is a medical emergency.

84. Can von Willebrand disease cause joint bleeds?

Von Willebrand disease predisposes to bleeding, including bleeding into the joints. Bleeding into the joints usually results from injury. The more severe the VWD, the less trauma is required to cause a joint bleed. People with hemophilia can have bleeding into the joints without any injury at all. They can have repeated bleeding into the same joint (a target joint), which can cause permanent damage, resulting in a joint that is painful and does not function properly. Spontaneous bleeding into the joints, however, is not usually a problem for people with VWD, except for those with severe disease and low factor VIII levels.

Vicki's story (type 3 VWD):

For the next few years after I was diagnosed with VWD, my parents dealt with constant trips to the emergency room for nosebleeds and gum bleeds. I traveled two and a half hours every three months to Boston Children's Hospital for clinic. By the time I was 4, I had started having bleeding into both of my ankle joints, with pain so intense that I could not tolerate the pressure of a bed sheet. My dad made a form for the end of the bed that lifted the sheet so it would not touch my feet.

By the age of 5, the doctors knew my ankles had deteriorated so much that the joint was concave and that I would need to be taken off my feet. Once I achieved full growth (around the age of 14) my ankles would need to be fused and there was the possibility that I would never walk. Orthopedics in Boston developed a pair of Patton bottom leg braces for me with my pelvic girdle supporting all my body weight. They looked like stilts, on a round pad of about four inches in diameter, and balanced my feet six inches off the ground. My feet were encased in ugly brown shoes that laced up over my ankles. The shoes were attached to the braces with a thick leather strap to keep my feet at a 90-degree angle. The braces did not bend. I used crutches to supplement walking but soon learned how to function without the crutches in most situations.

My dad again created a device that looked like a ramp for me to use in school that would allow my legs to rest and not hang down. I also had full leg casts made periodically to sleep in. These casts kept my feet at a 90-degree angle. I remember the doctors telling my mother to let me be a kid: if I fell, to let me pick myself up and get going again. This caused my mother to receive many comments from friends and family.

My mom found a Christian camp that would take me for a week as long as mom and dad were nearby. After a year or two this was not required, and I spent the next eight years attending this camp every summer. After four years of braces the doctors noticed some improvement and bone regeneration in the ankles and decided that I did not need full leg braces, and when I was age 10, they developed braces from the knee down. The pads were shaped more like a foot and allowed me to move more naturally.

At age 12, the doctors were amazed to find that my ankle joints had regrown to a more rounded shape from the extreme concave or total destruction that had necessitated the braces. I was free! I was walking for the first time in 6 years. I was able to shop for shoes, not being restricted any more to the orthopedic shoe used in the braces. I learned to ride a two-wheeled bike. Try being a kid on a full-sized tricycle!! I learned to square dance, participated in 4-H dress reviews, and began middle school as a "normal" kid. I still had nosebleeds, dealt with dental bleeds and bruises, but was nearly independent. My ankles acted up every now and then, but I worked retail, on my feet most of the time until I was 21.

Eventually, however, not only did I have a problem with my ankles, but I started having problems with my right elbow.

It was not until 1998 that I connected with a hematologist and the hemophilia treatment center in southern Maine. I figured that it had been six years since my last bleed (I dismissed the joint bleeds as commonplace), and I tended to have a bleed about every eight to ten years, so it was time that I indoctrinated a hematologist, just to be prepared. My first visit to clinic opened my eyes to the advances in treatment for bleeding disorders and that I was not alone. Do I still have bleeding issues? Yes, arthritis has settled into all six of my target joints, so I have difficulty recognizing a bleed. I treat when I am unsure. My ankles are back in braces because I have lost all cartilage and am rubbing bone on bone. My left has lost all movement and rotation and is fusing the joint together by itself; the right is not much better. We are hoping that both will fuse by themselves and I will avoid surgery down the road.

PART FIVE

Living with VWD

Are there medications that I should avoid?

Does eating foods high in vitamin K prevent bleeding?

Is a medical identification bracelet necessary?

More . . .

85. Does a person with VWD need any special vaccinations?

The vaccines that are recommended for all individuals are listed on the United States Centers for Disease Control and Prevention (CDC) Web site (www.cdc.gov/vaccines; see "Immunization Schedules"). Although the hepatitis A vaccine is recommended for everyone under age 2, and hepatitis B vaccine is recommended for everyone under age 18, individuals with VWD are more likely to require a transfusion and should be protected against viruses that could be transmitted by blood products or von Willebrand factor concentrates. Therefore, individuals with VWD should receive both the hepatitis A and hepatitis B vaccine series regardless of age. Although changes in clotting factor preparation practices and donor screening have greatly reduced the risk of an individual acquiring hepatitis A or B from clotting factors, the CDC still recommends that susceptible (nonimmunized) individuals be immunized against hepatitis A or B before the administration of clotting factors. Unfortunately, there is no vaccine against hepatitis C.

86. Are there medications that I should avoid?

Since many nonprescription products contain aspirin or aspirin-like medicines, you need to read labels carefully.

If you have VWD, you should consult your doctor before taking any new medications. You should generally avoid medications that increase the risk of bleeding. Aspirin and aspirin-like drugs inhibit platelets, reduce the ability of blood to clot, and can result in bleeding and therefore should be avoided. Since many nonprescription products contain aspirin or aspirin-like medicines, you need to read labels carefully. Nonsteroidal anti-inflammatory drugs (NSAIDs), such as ibuprofen and naproxen, inhibit platelets to a lesser degree but may still reduce the ability of blood to clot and may increase the risk of bleeding. The risk of bleeding is probably not great, so NSAIDs may still be prescribed to individuals with VWD for short periods of time to treat specific problems. Generally, however, you should avoid NSAIDs. Many nonprescription products contain ibuprofen or naproxen, so again, you should read labels carefully. For instance, Midol® comes in six different formulations; four do not contain an NSAID, but one contains ibuprofen and one contains naproxen.

Recently, certain antidepressants have been shown to increase the risk of bleeding. Many antidepressants are believed to work by blocking the natural chemical serotonin from entering other tissues and keeping more of it in the brain, where it can improve mood. These antidepressants are called selective serotonin reuptake inhibitors, or SSRIs. Platelets use serotonin to help them stick to one another or aggregate. By blocking serotonin from entering platelets, many antidepressants have the potential to reduce the levels of serotonin in platelets, suppress their ability to function, and increase the risk of bleeding. In individuals without a bleeding disorder, the risk of bleeding is about 1 percent. Even in individuals with a bleeding disorder, the risk of bleeding is probably not great. Nonetheless, there are antidepressant medications that do not have the same effect on serotonin and do not carry the same risk of bleeding. These medications could be tried first.

Even in individuals with a bleeding disorder, anticoagulant medications (such as heparin and warfarin) and antiplatelet medications (such as aspirin, dipyridamole, clopidogrel, and ticlodipine) may be necessary to treat abnormal blood clots (see Question 49). An individual with VWD, however, should take anticoagulant

An individual with VWD, however, should take anticoagulant or antiplatelet medications only with the blessing of a hematologist.

or antiplatelet medications only with the blessing of a hematologist. Medications that increase the risk of bleeding are summarized in **Table 1**.

Andra's story (low VWF or mild type 1 VWD):

I like relief when I am in pain, but I do not like the fuzzy-headed feeling I get after taking narcotic pain relievers. After my hysterectomy, I was offered Toradol® so that I would not have to take narcotic pain relievers. What was I thinking? I must have been fuzzy-headed! I took the Toradol®, which I now believe contributed to my postoperative complications. I had bleeding into my wound and then it became infected. I needed a second surgery, three weeks of intravenous antibiotics, and six weeks of dressing changes. I am a doctor. You would think I would know better than to take a medication that could inhibit my platelets.

87. What medications are safe to take for pain relief?

If you have VWD, you should consult your doctor about what medications are safe to take for pain relief. Tylenol® (acetaminophen) is a pain reliever that does not increase the risk of bleeding and is generally considered safe. Celebrex® is an NSAID (nonsteroidal anti-inflammatory drug) that is just as effective at relieving pain and inflammation as ibuprofen and naproxen but has a lower risk of bleeding. Celebrex® is not prescribed as often as it used to be because it may increase the risk of heart attacks in susceptible people. Vioxx®, a similar NSAID, was taken off of the market for that reason. Narcotic medications such as codeine, oxycodone (the narcotic in Percocet®), and hydrocodone (the narcotic in Vicodin®) have no effect on platelets and are safe to take.

Table 1

Brand Name of Drug	Generic Name	Reason Taken	Possible Problems
Advil®	ibuprofen	To relieve pain and inflammation.	See ibuprofen.
Aleve®	naproxen	To relieve pain and inflammation.	See naproxen.
Alka-Seltzer®	contains aspirin, sodium bicarbonate, and citric acid	To treat heartburn, indigestion, and headache.	See aspirin.
Anacin®	aspirin and caffeine	To relieve pain and inflammation.	See aspirin.
Anafranil®	clomipramine	To treat obsessive–compulsive disorder.	Lowers levels of serotonin in platelets, reduces platelet function to some degree, may reduce the ability of blood to clot, and may increase the risk of bleeding.
	aspirin	To relieve pain and inflammation.	Inhibits platelets, reduces the ability of blood to clot, and can result in bleeding.
BC® Powder	contains aspirin, acetaminophen (the generic version of Tylenol®), and caffeine	To relieve pain and inflammation.	See aspirin.
Bufferin®	aspirin	To relieve pain and inflammation.	See aspirin.
Celexa®	citalopram	To treat depression.	See SSRIs.
Coumadin®	warfarin	To treat abnormal blood clots.	See warfarin.
Darvon-65®	contains propoxyphene, aspirin, and caffeine	To relieve pain and inflammation.	See aspirin.
Doan's Pills®	Contains magnesium salicylate (an aspirin-like drug) and diphenhydramine (the generic version of Bendadryl®)	To relieve pain and inflammation.	See aspirin.
Ecotrin®	aspirin	To relieve pain and inflammation.	See aspirin.
Effexor®	venlafaxine	To treat depression.	Blocks reuptake of norepinephrine and serotonin. See SSRIs.
Empirin®	contains aspirin	To relieve pain and inflammation.	See aspirin.
Excedrin®	contains aspirin, acetaminophen (the generic version of Tylenol®), and caffeine	To relieve pain and inflammation.	See aspirin.
Fragmin®	dalteparin (a longer-acting form of heparin)	To treat abnormal blood clots.	See heparin.
Goody's Powder®	contains aspirin, acetaminophen (the generic version of Tylenol®), and caffeine	To relieve pain and inflammation.	See aspirin.

(continues) 93

Table 1 (continued)

Brand Name of Drug	Generic Name	Reason Taken	Possible Problems
	heparin	To treat abnormal blood clots.	Prevents blood from clotting and can cause bleeding.
	ibuprofen	To relieve pain and inflammation.	Inhibits platelets to some degree, and, therefore, may somewhat reduce the ability of blood to clot and may increase the risk of bleeding.
Lexapro®	citalopram	To treat anxiety and depression.	See SSRIs.
Lovenox®	enoxaparin (a longer-acting form of heparin)	To treat abnormal blood clots.	See heparin.
Midol® Cramps & Body Aches	ibuprofen	To relieve pain and inflammation.	See ibuprofen.
Midol® Cramps & Body Aches	naproxen	To relieve pain and inflammation.	See naproxen.
Motrin®	ibuprofen	To relieve pain and inflammation.	See ibuprofen.
	naproxen	To relieve pain and inflammation.	Inhibits platelets to some degree, and, therefore, may somewhat reduce the ability of blood to clot and may increase the risk of bleeding.
Paxil®	paroxetine	To treat depression.	See SSRIs.
Pepto-Bismol®	contains bismuth subsalicylate (an aspirin-like drug)	To treat nausea, heartburn, upset stomach, indigestion, and diarrhea.	See aspirin.
Persantine®	dipyridamole	To prevent blood clots from forming on replaced heart valves and to prevent heart attack.	Inhibits platelets and can cause bleeding.
Plavix®	clopidogrel	To prevent heart attack and stroke.	Inhibits platelets and can cause bleeding.
Prozac®	fluoxetine	To treat depression.	See SSRIs.
	serotonin reuptake inhibitors or SSRIs	A category of drugs used to treat depression.	Lowers levels of serotonin in platelets, reduces platelet function to some degree, may reduce the ability of blood to clot, and may increase the risk of bleeding.
Ticlid®	ticlodipine	To prevent heart attack and stroke.	Inhibits platelets and can cause bleeding.
Toradol®	ketorolac	To treat pain in the hospital.	Inhibits platelets and can cause bleeding.
	warfarin	To treat abnormal blood clots.	Prevents blood from clotting and can cause bleeding.
Zoloft®	sertraline	To treat depression.	See SSRIs.

Garry's story (type 2A von Willebrand disease):

Last year I was taking ibuprofen three times a week when I began to have bleeding in my eyes. I stopped the ibuprofen! Now I take Celebrex®.

88. Are there antidepressant medications that do not affect platelets?

As described in Question 86, many antidepressants are believed to work by blocking the natural chemical serotonin from entering tissues other than the brain. By blocking serotonin from entering platelets, these medications have the potential to reduce platelet function and increase the risk of bleeding. There are antidepressant medications that do not have the same effect on serotonin and do not carry the same bleeding risk. These medications include doxepin, Remeron® (mirtazapine), and Wellbutrin® (buproprion).

89. Are there natural remedies that prevent bleeding?

There are natural remedies that are advertised to prevent bleeding, but none is recognized by the medical profession to prevent bleeding.

90. Are there natural remedies that should be avoided?

Not much is known about dietary supplements and herbal medications and their interaction with von Willebrand disease, but some may increase the risk of bleeding and are best avoided. They are summarized in **Table 2**.

Table 2

Herbal Medication or Dietary Supplement	Reason Taken	Possible Problems
Arnica	To treat bruises, sprains, inflammation, and bleeding at the time of surgery.	May cause bleeding at the time of surgery.
Bilberry	To treat diarrhea, minor mucus membrane inflammation, and a variety of eye disorders, including poor night vision, eyestrain, and myopia (nearsightedness).	In large doses, increases the risk of bleeding.
Bromelain	To assist in the digestion of proteins and to treat inflammation of the nose and sinuses.	May increase the risk of bleeding.
Cat's claw	To treat the pain and inflammation of arthritis and to boost the immune system.	May increase the risk of bleeding.
Coenzyme Q10	To increase health in chronic diseases.	May lower platelets and, therefore, increase the risk of bleeding.
Coleus (forskolin)	To treat various heart and lung ailments.	May increase the risk of bleeding.
Danshen (Salvia miltiorrhiza)	To treat circulatory disorders.	Suppresses platelet function and increases the risk of bleeding.
Dong Quai (Chinese Angelica)	To treat menopausal symptoms, premenstrual syndrome, irregular menstrual cycles.	May affect clotting factors and platelets and increase the risk of bleeding.
Feverfew	To treat headaches.	Increases bleeding.
Garlic	To decrease cholesterol and blood clot formation.	Suppresses platelet function and increases the risk of bleeding.
Ginger	To relieve nausea.	Suppresses platelet function and may increase the risk of bleeding.
Ginkgo biloba	To improve circulation, especially to the brain; also to prevent memory loss, dizziness, and headaches.	Causes bleeding.
Ginseng	To increase energy and reduce stress.	May cause bleeding.
Horse chestnut	To treat chronic venous insufficiency, a condition that includes leg swelling, varicose veins, leg pain, itching, and skin ulcers.	May increase the risk of bleeding.
Pau d'arco	To treat a variety of chronic diseases.	Interferes with blood clotting and causes bleeding.
Red clover	To treat postmenopausal symptoms.	May increase the risk of bleeding.
Sweet clover (melilot)	To treat chronic venous insufficiency and phlebitis.	Contains substances related to the blood thinner warfarin (Coumadin®) and causes bleeding.
Sweet woodruff	To treat inflammation and constipation. To flavor May wines and some foods.	Contains substances related to the blood thinner warfarin (Coumadin®) and in large amounts can cause bleeding.
Turmeric	To treat stomach and intestinal ailments and arthritis pain.	May increase the risk of bleeding.
Vitamin E	To lower cholesterol and boost the immune system.	High doses may increase the risk of bleeding.

91. Is it safe to eat garlic?

The amount of garlic used to flavor food does not interfere with platelet function, does not increase the risk of bleeding, and is safe to eat.

92. Are there any other foods that I should avoid?

If you are severely affected and have experienced mouth bleeds, you may want to avoid foods with sharp edges that could cause cuts in the mouth and very hot foods that could burn the tongue or roof of the mouth.

93. Does vitamin C prevent bleeding?

In a person with a normal, balanced diet, vitamin C does not prevent bleeding, but deficiency of vitamin C, a disease known as scurvy, can cause bleeding. Like other vitamins, vitamin C is an essential molecule that comes from natural sources, but humans do not make vitamin C for themselves. It is necessary for the formation of collagen, a protein that accounts for one-third of the body's total protein. Collagen provides structure to blood vessels. Normal collagen is necessary for von Willebrand factor to adhere platelets to subendothelium (the tissue below the lining or endothelium of blood vessels). In scurvy, or vitamin C deficiency, abnormal collagen prevents normal platelet adhesion and can result in bleeding symptoms not unlike those of VWD.

In scurvy, or vitamin C deficiency, abnormal collagen prevents normal platelet adhesion and can result in bleeding symptoms not unlike those of VWD.

Scurvy can be prevented by a diet that includes certain citrus fruits such as oranges or lemons. Other foods rich in vitamin C are fruits such as black currants, guava, kiwi, papaya, tomatoes, and strawberries. It can also be found in some vegetables, such as bell peppers, broccoli, potatoes, cabbage, spinach, and paprika, as well as some pickled vegetables. A normal, balanced diet contains adequate vitamin C, and therefore supplements are not necessary. Multiple vitamins, however, do contain vitamin C. Vitamin C is destroyed by pasteurization, so infant formula is supplemented with vitamin C. Breast milk contains adequate vitamin C if the mother's diet contains sufficient vitamin C. Scurvy is rare in North America or Europe, but it can still occur in individuals with a diet devoid of fresh fruits and vegetables or vitamin supplements.

94. Does eating foods high in vitamin K prevent bleeding?

Vitamin K is essential to the liver's production of the active forms of several clotting factors. Vitamin K may have a role in bone health, but its most important role is in blood clotting. Like other vitamins, vitamin K is an essential molecule that comes from natural sources, but humans do not make vitamin K for themselves. Humans get it from two sources, from what is produced by intestinal bacteria and from food. Unless people are deficient in vitamin K, there is no scientific evidence that eating more vitamin K–rich foods will improve blood clotting.

95. What about wine, beer, and liquor?

Excessive alcohol consumption can suppress platelet function; liver damage from chronic excessive alcohol consumption can reduce the body's production of clotting factors; driving while intoxicated can dramatically increase the risk of severe injury and bleeding; but wine, beer, and liquor in moderation probably do not increase the risk of bleeding.

96. What about exercise?

Physical activity is important for everyone, but especially for people with bleeding disorders. Exercise can help build stronger muscles, maintain flexibility, prevent joint damage, and improve venous access. Sports and exercise can also help build self-confidence, teach teamwork, and create a sense of community. Precautions that people with bleeding disorders should take include stretching before exercise and wearing helmets, wrist, and knee protection when appropriate.

97. What about sports?

Some sports such as swimming, biking, and walking are considered safe for everyone. Other sports such as football, hockey, wrestling, and lifting heavy weights are not considered safe activities for people with moderate or severe VWD. Recommendations concerning which sports are appropriate must be individualized. Most people with mild VWD will be able to engage in any sport, while people with moderate or severe VWD should probably avoid contact sports and sports that carry a higher risk of injury. Below is a list of some specific sports and activities, classified according to their risk of injury that could lead to bleeding.

Sports that carry a very low risk of injury are:

> Archery
> Elliptical machines
> Fishing
> Frisbee
> Golf
> Hiking
> Tai chi
> Sailing
> Snorkeling

Physical activity is important for everyone, but especially for people with bleeding disorders.

Stationary biking
Swimming
Walking
Water exercises

Sports that still carry a relatively low risk of injury include:

Bicycling
Body sculpting
Physioball
Pilates
Rowing machine
Spinning
Treadmill
Weight lifting and resistance training

Sports that carry some risk of injury include:

Aerobics
Bowling
Cardio kickboxing
Cross-country skiing
Dance
Jogging or running
Rock climbing
Roller skating or rollerblading
Rowing or crew
T-ball
Tennis
Ultimate Frisbee
Yoga

Sports that carry a moderate risk of injury and should be avoided by people with severe VWD include:

Baseball and softball
Basketball
Canoeing, kayaking, or river rafting
Cheerleading

Downhill skiing

Gymnastics

Horseback riding

Ice skating

Jet skiing

Karate, kung fu, tae kwon do

Mountain biking

Racquetball

Scuba diving

Skateboarding

Snowboarding

Soccer

Surfing

Track and field

Volleyball

Waterskiing

Sports that carry a high risk of injury and should be avoided not only by people with moderate or severe VWD, but also by people with mild VWD (or anyone else who wants to avoid spending time in an emergency room):

BMX racing

Boxing

Competitive diving

Football

Hockey (field hockey or ice hockey)

Lacrosse

Motorcycling or motocross racing

Power lifting

Rock climbing (outdoors)

Rodeo

Rugby

Snowmobiling

Trampoline

Weight lifting or power training

Wrestling

Ray's story (type 1 VWD with moderate bleeding problems):

I was first diagnosed when I was 3 years old. I was undergoing a pre-op evaluation prior to having an adenoidectomy, and the routine pre-op labs showed an abnormal aPTT test.

I have since learned that it is unusual to have a prolonged aPTT, but if the aPTT test had not been prolonged, I am not sure when I would have been diagnosed. In retrospect, I had had symptoms sooner. My mother tells me that I bruised easily and once, when I was 18 months old, I fell and cut my eye on the corner of a speaker. It oozed for three days.

I was always active playing ball when I was little. After I was diagnosed, my parents decided to allow me to be as involved in sports as I wanted with the limitations of contact sports like tackle football. They felt the stronger my muscles were, the better protected my joints would become. They also thought different sports would assist in my developing good coordination and agility. I have participated in a number of sports since then. These include:

> *Gymnastics—ages 3–5*
> *Baseball—ages 5–12*
> *Karate—starting at age 8 and continuing*
> *Track and field—7th–12th grade*
> *Deck hockey—pick up games starting in high school and continuing*
> *Volleyball—starting in 9th grade on a recreation league and continuing*
> *Swimming—starting as a sophomore in high school and continuing in college*
> *Cross-country—12th grade*
> *Intramural basketball—starting in high school and continuing*
> *Flag football—starting in high school and continuing*
> *Ultimate Frisbee—starting in college and continuing*

I've had to take some precautions. I avoid contact sports. When I played baseball as a child, I wore a protective vest. Some of the parents liked the idea and would borrow it for their sons. As I got older and grew out of the vests, the only option was to go to a Kevlar® (bullet-proof vest), which was heavy. That is the age I stopped playing organized baseball. When I was ages 12 to 17, I had a series of injuries, including a stress fracture of my ankle, sprained ankles, and hip bleeds. I was extremely active and growing a lot during this period of time in my life. As a consequence, I started using prophylaxis against bleeding with DDAVP (Stimate®). Fortunately, I have not had any repetitive motion bleeding. There were a lot of times I had to be treated with intravenous (IV) DDAVP over two to three days. In 2005, I started college. In the spring of 2006, I tore three tendons. The doctor at the hemophilia treatment center was concerned about the amount of bleeding I was having and recommended Humate-P®. It worked extremely well. I have always been thankful for the physicians I have. When I am home or at college, I have the assurance that my doctors are not only very knowledgeable but always available via the telephone or through the hospital.

I pre-treat before some sporting events. For instance, I pre-treat prior to a karate tournament. If I am skeptical that I am having a bleed, I treat. Most of my bleeds do not occur immediately after an injury. I had to learn to be aware of my symptoms with bleeds. My bleeds usually occur 24 to 48 hours later. When I travel, I don't always take my Stimate® with me. If it is a sporting event I am participating in, I take it with me just in case. I also know where treatment centers are when I travel. I do not use Stimate® daily, weekly, or even monthly. I do use it prior to dental procedures. I had minor surgery (removal of cysts) last year and used IV DDAVP with success.

I became involved in the bleeding disorders community at age 11. I began to attend meetings and attended camps for people with bleeding disorders. The first camp I attended was Camp Horseshoe in West Virginia and later attended Camp Hot-To-Clot in Erie, PA. I have learned a lot at these camps and also it was a great way to be very adventurous in a safe way. Everyone there has the same issues and we could share and learn from each other. Recently, I have become involved with a program called "Gettin' in the Game," a program sponsored by CSL Behring that encourages safe participation in sports.

With respect to my bleeding disorder, I find it extremely important to be pro-active, not re-active. By this, I mean that I have the mentality of what I can do, even though I have a bleeding disorder, rather than the mentality of what can't I do, because I have a bleeding disorder. Even with this mindset, I am prepared. When an injury occurs, I stop my activities, seek treatment, rest the bleed area, follow up with any necessary therapy, and after proper healing has occurred, begin activities again. I also learned to play the guitar and chess, so when I have downtimes from bleeds, I still have something to do. It also passes the time and takes my mind off the treatment when I am being infused. I continue to train and play sports for two reasons. The first is my love for sports of all kinds. The second is to keep in top condition so as to prevent injuries. My motto is "the harder I train, the harder I can play."

People with moderate or severe disease should anticipate the possibility of requiring treatment while they are away from home.

98. What about travel?

People with VWD can travel wherever they please. People with moderate or severe disease should anticipate the possibility of requiring treatment while they are away from home. They should know their type of VWD and their exact prescription for DDAVP, von Willebrand factor concentrates, or other medications that they use. They should have the contact information for their hematologist or hemophilia treatment center and they should know where hemophilia treatment centers are en route and at their destination. People with VWD who self-infuse VWF concentrate should take a sufficient supply of VWF concentrate with them, as well as a sufficient supply of needles and syringes. People who do not self-infuse may still want to talk to their hematologist or nurse coordinator at their hemophilia treatment center about carrying DDAVP or VWF concentrate with them, since these products are not available everywhere. A cooler may be necessary to keep products at the right temperature. People with VWD might want to make sure that their insurance policy will cover any necessary medical care while away from home. Travel insurance may be an option if one's regular policy does not provide coverage.

International travelers should consult **Passport**, a directory of international hemophilia treatment centers. Passport can be found on the World Federation of Hemophilia Web site (www.wfh.org), under Resources. Travelers can use the various search features to get a list of hemophilia treatment centers in various countries and to find a specific organization or person.

99. Is a medical identification bracelet necessary?

Wearing a medical identification bracelet or necklace is an excellent idea for a person with a serious bleeding disorder, such as moderate or severe VWD. Such an identifier should be worn continuously and can alert emergency medical personnel that a person has a significant risk of bleeding. Emergency medical personnel

Wearing a medical identification bracelet or necklace is an excellent idea for a person with a serious bleeding disorder, such as moderate or severe VWD.

do pay attention to such jewelry. "von Willebrand disease" can be engraved on the surface of this bracelet or necklace. In addition, any other information that would be important in an emergency—such as recommended treatment in the case of bleeding, medications, other medical conditions, and allergies—should be engraved there as well. Emergency contacts (next of kin, physician) and other information can be included as space permits. Additional information can be carried on a card in a wallet or purse. As a precaution, an individual's physician or other health care provider should approve what will be engraved on the medical identification tag. Order forms can be obtained from a health care provider's office or can be downloaded from the Internet.

Vicki's story (type 3 VWD):

I had started wearing a MedicAlert® bracelet prior to adopting our daughter. This had been a requirement of the adoption agency, but something I had never done before, because I thought I was the only person with VWD and no one would know what to do with me in an emergency situation anyway. So, once I had been told about the VWF/FVIII concentrates, I dutifully added the information about my type of VWD and [the VWF/FVIII concentrates] to my bracelet and continued my life.

Jessica's story (type 1 VWD):

I wear a medical identification bracelet; it's engraved with "von Willebrand" as well as my medication allergy. I was reluctant to wear one at first because I thought it would be an unattractive advertisement about my VWD, but I went to a local jeweler and worked with them to pick out something that I love. They ordered the MedicAlert® "plate" separately, and I picked out a bracelet chain out of the jeweler's selection, so I wasn't limited to the preset combinations I had found at other places. As trivial as it may seem, it was important to me to have something that blended with my personal style rather than call more attention to my VWD.

Karen's story (husband and daughters with type 2B VWD):

My husband, who has type 2B VWD, has always worn a MedicAlert® necklace, as did his dad, since their diagnoses. So when the girls got diagnosed, I ordered MedicAlert® bracelets and put them on their little ankles.

Of course the primary reason for their MedicAlert®s was so their information would be on file in case of an emergency. However, the secondary reason was so I didn't get turned in for child abuse! They always were bruised and I had more than one occasion when I was questioned because of their bruising. I do have to say, I never took offense at that—I appreciated that people, even strangers, were watching out for children's welfare and safety.

Now fast forward. (I have permission to share this.) Steph got to be a teenager and she decided she didn't want to wear her MedicAlert® anymore. She hated people asking her what it was for. She didn't like being different.

We are very close, and one rainy afternoon when she was a freshman in high school we had one of the biggest disagreements we ever had. We were in the car driving during a miserable (and potentially dangerous) thunderstorm when I found out she didn't have her MedicAlert® on. It scared the daylights out of me. I punished her for not wearing it (she didn't get to go to a movie with friends she had been looking forward to). And since she was a good kid, I thought that was the end of it.

But she continued not to wear her MedicAlert®. I tried everything. I got custom-made jewelry with her info on it (they didn't have any attractive MedicAlert®s like they do now). I begged. I pleaded. I knew she had her MedicAlert® card in her wallet but in an accident, she might get separated from her purse. Every time we talked about it, we got into a huge fight. It is the only thing we have ever really fought about.

She is now 22, a senior in college, and she doesn't live at home anymore. She still will not wear a MedicAlert®.

Now I'm baring my soul here but I confess that I always have this deep, nagging (not really on the surface) fear that she will be in an accident and she will bleed out. I know wearing a MedicAlert® isn't a guarantee that she would be fine, but at least medical personnel would be aware that she has a bleeding disorder.

As a mom, a car accident is my greatest fear. That said, my faith is strong and I know worrying doesn't help. But if I'm honest, the worry is there, particularly when she is driving. I am resigned to the fact that she is an adult and she has to make her own decisions and choices. I also know it is the only subject that is such a "hot potato" that we can't even begin to discuss it. But I will always be her mother.

I know that she doesn't remember those nights when she was little and I held her while she bled all night long. She doesn't know how hard it is to watch your screaming child get medical procedures that are painful, but necessary. She doesn't know what it is like to lie in bed at night waiting for her to call and check in and let me know she is okay.

But I don't know what it is like to be in her shoes.

Maybe when she has her own children, she'll understand. But until that time, I try to respect her and be there for when she needs me. I pray every night that God will protect and watch over her. And that is all I know how to do.

100. Where can I get more information?

The Appendix that follows includes a list of resources that individuals with VWD and their families may find useful.

Appendix

Resources

All About Bleeding

www.allaboutbleeding.com

All About Bleeding is an online resource dedicated to increasing awareness about VWD. Although the Web site www.allaboutbleeding.com is sponsored by the CSL Behring company, it contains no advertising. The Web site has information for people with VWD. People with VWD can also share their stories and ask questions of an expert.

Canadian Hemophilia Society

www.hemophilia.ca

The Canadian Hemophilia Society serves people with inherited bleeding disorders. These bleeding disorders include hemophilia, VWD, rare factor deficiencies, and platelet disorders. The Canadian Hemophilia Society is an organization that works at three levels: nationally, provincially, and locally. They have ten provincial chapters across the country. Some of the chapters have additional local structures that they refer to as regions. Together, they form the Canadian Hemophilia Society. Their Web site contains clear, accurate information about VWD.

The National Heart, Lung, and Blood Institute (NHLBI) of the National Institute of Health (NIH)

www.nhlbi.nih.gov

The NHLBI von Willebrand Disease Expert Panel was established in spring 2004 in response to a recommendation from the fiscal year 2004 Congressional Appropriations Conference Committee. The committee urged the NHLBI to work with medical associations and experts in the field to develop a set of treatment guidelines for VWD. On February 29, 2008, the NHLBI issued the first clinical guidelines for the diagnosis and management of VWD to be published in the United States. The guidelines include recommendations on screening, diagnosis, disease management, and directions for future research. In addition to the guidelines, the NHLBI has developed a pocket guide for physicians as well as a fact sheet for patients and the public. More information about VWD, and the fact sheet, can be found on the NHLBI Web site.

The National Hemophilia Foundation (NHF)
www.hemophilia.org

The NHF is an organization dedicated to finding better treatments and cures for bleeding and clotting disorders and preventing the complications of these disorders through education, advocacy, and research. Established in 1948, the NHF is a nonprofit 501(c)3 organization with chapters throughout the United States. Its programs and initiatives are made possible through the generosity of individuals, corporations, and foundations as well as through a cooperative agreement with the Centers for Disease Control and Prevention (CDC). Once a year in the fall, the NHF holds its annual meeting. Approximately 3,000 people attend this meeting, including individuals with bleeding disorders, family members, health care providers, and employees of companies that provide products and services to people with bleeding disorders. More information can be found on the NHF Web site. Once or twice a year the NHF works with a state or local chapter of the organization and takes a program "On the Road" outside of New York City.

While the NHF's headquarters are in New York City, the NHF is also organized into a network of local or state chapters. On the NHF home page, there is a link to the Chapter Center Web page, which, in turn, links to Web pages for local and state chapters. Local and state chapters can put individuals in touch with other people with VWD who can provide advice and information. Additionally, local and state chapters hold informational meetings and social events.

Vicki's story (type 3 VWD):

I was 40 years old before I finally had something to control my bleeding. I considered myself a relatively educated woman, but I was totally in the dark concerning my bleeding disorder. Throughout the next year I began researching bleeding disorders, found out that I was not so different from people with other bleeding deficiencies, and also found out that VWD was the most common bleeding disorder, yet the least diagnosed. I attended our local hemophilia chapter's family camp and met other bleeders for the first time.

I also learned at family camp to self-infuse. My intent at first was just normal curiosity and to learn how to mix the factor. When asked to attend a women's retreat in New York City, I decided that I needed to be able to infuse myself and not depend on others. After all, if the 10- and 12-year-old boys at camp could do infusions, then by hokey, so could I!! At this retreat I met other women with bleeding disorders and truly became part of a community. Since then, I have attended many events locally and nationally to network with others with bleeding disorders. I now work for the New England Hemophilia Association and provide programs for Maine members and coordinate the Project Red Flag initiative in New England by raising the awareness of women with bleeding disorders within the health care community.

Jeanette's story (type 1 VWD with a platelet defect):

I recently have become active on the part of women with bleeding disorders. I am an educated and successful business-woman, but I haven't known as much as I could have known about my bleeding disorder. For instance, it wasn't until a year ago that I learned that insurance will pay for VWF concentrates and that they can be self-infused. I am trying to learn as much as possible and am trying to take better care of myself. How else can I help my children, especially my daughters?

Project Red Flag is the National Hemophilia Foundation's (NHF) public awareness campaign to reach the estimated two and a half million women in the United States with undiagnosed bleeding disorders. The campaign educates women, their health care providers, and policy makers about the symptoms of bleeding disorders, especially VWD, and encourages proper diagnosis and treatment. NHF has developed many resources that are available as part of the Project Red Flag campaign. Project Red Flag resources have been designed to help NHF chapters, hemophilia treatment centers, and consumers raise awareness of women's bleeding disorders in their local communities. Some of these resources can be obtained through the NHF's information service, HANDI. More information is available on the NHF Web site.

HANDI is the NHF's information service. Since 1991, HANDI has grown into a full-fledged resource center for people with bleeding disorders. Its primary objective is to answer consumer's questions; HANDI provides quality educational publications, makes referrals to additional sources of assistance, and responds to the needs of individuals and organizations. HANDI processes requests for information from a wide variety of individuals and organizations including NHF chapters, medical professionals, consumers and their families, and teachers and students conducting research. The types of information requested reflect a diversity of needs—topics include areas of particular interest to people with VWD, such as self-infusion of clotting factor concentrates, psychosocial issues, women's health, and financial and insurance reimbursement issues. HANDI's current resource collection contains more than 12,000 items including article reprints, textbooks, educational publications, CD-ROMs, and videos. HANDI staff members are available Monday through Friday, 9 AM to 5:30 PM EST, to answer questions. They can be reached at 1-800-42HANDI or via e-mail at handi@hemophilia.org. Requests can also be faxed to (212) 328-3799.

United States Centers for Disease Control and Prevention (CDC) Division of Blood Disorders

www.cdc.gov/ncbddd/hbd/about_hbd.htm

The CDC Division of Blood Disorders collaborates with health care providers, university medical centers, community-based organizations, and national and international preventive health agencies to implement specialized prevention programs for persons with blood disorders, including VWD. Currently, the Division of Blood Disorders has four key goals:

- enhance blood safety to prevent the transmission of infectious diseases to persons being treated with blood products
- identify risk factors through evidence-based research and surveillance and implement interventions to prevent complications of blood disorders

- prevent and reduce complications of bleeding and clotting disorders that specifically affect women's health
- develop and deliver consistent prevention education messages to encourage affected persons to make informed decisions about their own health care.

A key activity involves collaborating with networks of specialized health care centers, including hemophilia treatment centers (HTCs) throughout the United States. A directory of hemophilia treatment centers can be found on the Division of Blood Disorders Web site. The Web site also has information about bleeding disorders, including VWD.

The World Federation of Hemophilia (WFH)

www.wfh.org

The World Federation of Hemophilia (WFH) was established in 1963 by Frank Schnabel, a Montreal businessman born with severe hemophilia A. His vision was to improve treatment and care for "the hundreds of thousands of hemophiliacs" worldwide through a new international organization. From a base of six national hemophilia societies, the Federation grew rapidly. It holds world congresses every two years and has created a global network of health care providers, national hemophilia associations, and people with hemophilia and their families. The WFH reached a turning point in 1969 when the World Health Organization acknowledged the Federation's growing international reputation and established official relations. The two bodies began working on joint projects.

Information about VWD can be found on the WFH Web site.

Glossary

A

Activated partial thromboplastin time (aPTT): A blood test that measures the length of time (in seconds) that it takes for clotting to occur when certain substances are added to the plasma or liquid portion of blood in a test tube.

Antifibrinolytic: A medication that can reduce the risk of bleeding by preventing normal blood clots that have formed at the site of blood vessel injury from being broken down or lysed.

Autosomal dominant transmission: The mode of inheritance when there is an abnormal gene on one of the chromosomes among the 22 pairs of autosomes, or non–sex (X or Y) chromosomes. Only one of the parents will have the condition caused by the abnormal gene. Only one parent needs to have the abnormal gene for the condition to be transmitted.

Autosomal recessive transmission: The mode of inheritance when there is an abnormal gene on both chromosomes in a pair of the 22 pairs of autosomes, or non–sex (X or Y) chromosomes.

B

Blood: A fluid that transports essential substances around the body, and is composed of water, proteins, other molecules, and cells.

Blood vessels: Tubes that carry blood to organs and extremities.

C

Clot: A plug of platelets and other cells held in place by a fibrin net that prevents blood from leaking out of an injured blood vessel.

Clotting factor: A specialized protein that is essential to prevent bleeding.

Complete blood count (CBC): A test for determining if anemia is present and how severe the anemia is and for determining if thrombocytopenia (an insufficient number of platelets) is present.

Cryoprecipitate: A product rich in factor VIII, fibrinogen, and von Willebrand factor (VWF) that is created from plasma by freezing it, slowly thawing it, then finally centrifuging it (a process that separates it by spinning it at very high speeds).

D

DDAVP: Also known as desmopressin, DDAVP is a synthetic version of the hormone vasopressin, which raises von Willebrand factor (VWF) levels by causing VWF to be released from the endothelial cells that line blood vessels.

Dysmenorrhea: Painful menstruation.

E

Endometriosis: The presence of patches of endometrial tissue, the tissue that lines the uterus, in the abdomen.

Endothelium: The lining of blood vessels.

F

Factor VIII: One of the clotting factors that is essential to prevent bleeding.

Fibrin: A solid mesh or net formed from fibrinogen, a specialized protein or clotting factor. Fibrin holds platelets and other cells in place and prevents blood from leaking out of an injured blood vessel.

Fresh frozen plasma (FFP): Plasma frozen shortly after being obtained from donors to preserve the clotting factors.

H

Hematologist: A doctor who is a specialist in the field of medicine that involves the study and treatment of blood disorders.

Hemoglobin: The molecule in the red blood cells that carries oxygen in the blood and gives blood its red color.

Hemophilia: A severe bleeding disorder that results from a deficiency of clotting factor VIII (hemophilia A) or clotting factor IX (hemophilia B).

Hemophilia treatment center (HTC): A clinic where a team of doctors, nurses, social workers, physical therapists, and other specialists work together to deliver comprehensive, state-of-the-art care to people with bleeding disorders.

M

Menorrhagia: Heavy menstrual bleeding.

P

Plasma: The liquid portion of blood that contains proteins and other molecules, but does not include cells.

PFA-100®: An automated test of platelet function.

Postpartum hemorrhage: Excessive bleeding after childbirth.

Platelets: The cells that prevent blood from leaking out of injured blood vessels.

Prothrombin time (PT): A blood test that measures the length of time (in seconds) that it takes for clotting to occur when tissue factor and other substances are added to the liquid portion of blood in a test tube.

S

Subendothelium: The tissue under the endothelium, which is the lining of the blood vessels. Platelets, the cells that prevent blood from leaking out of an injured blood vessel, stick or adhere to the subendothelium.

T

Topical agents: Medications that can be applied directly to tissue to stop bleeding.

V

von Willebrand disease (VWD): A bleeding tendency resulting from insufficient or low levels of von Willebrand, abnormal von Willebrand factor, or absent von Willebrand factor.

von Willebrand factor (VWF): A protein that is essential for normal blood clotting. It acts like a glue to stick or adhere platelets to the subendothelium at the site of blood vessel injury.

von Willebrand factor antigen (VWF: Ag): A test that measures the actual amount of von Willebrand factor (VWF) protein in a patient's plasma.

von Willebrand factor concentrate: A product purified from human plasma that is rich in von Willebrand factor.

von Willebrand factor multimers: Strings of von Willebrand subunits that form the active forms of von Willebrand factor.

von Willebrand ristocetin cofactor activity (VWF:RCo): A test that measures the function of von Willebrand factor (VWF).

Index